Feeding and Nutrition in Children with Neurodevelopmental Disability

Feeding and Nutrition in Children with Neurodevelopmental Disability

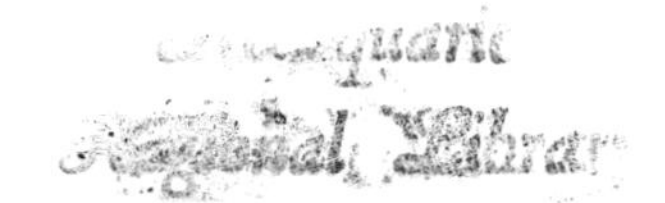

Edited by Peter B Sullivan

2009
Mac Keith Press
Distributed by Wiley-Blackwell

Editor: Hilary M. Hart
Managing Director, Mac Keith Press: Caroline Black
Project Manager: Annalisa Welch
Indexer: Dr Laurence Errington

First published in this edition 2009 by
Mac Keith Press, 6 Market Road, London N7 9PW, UK

British Library Cataloguing-in-Publication data
A catalogue record of this book is available from the British Library

ISBN: 978–1-898683–60–5

Typeset by Keystroke, 28 High Street, Tettenhall, Wolverhampton
Printed by The Lavenham Press Ltd, Water Street, Lavenham, Suffolk
Mac Keith Press is supported by Scope

Contents

Contributors

Wee Meng Han, Senior Dietitian, Department of Nutrition and Dietetics, KK Women's and Children's Hospital (formerly Paediatric Dietitian, The Children's Hospital, John Radcliffe Hospital, Oxford, UK)

Bridget R Lambert, Paediatric Dietitian, The Children's Hospital, John Radcliffe Hospital, Oxford, UK

Natalie A McKaig, Paediatric Dietitian, Department of Nutrition and Dietetics, Ninewells Hospital, Dundee, UK

Astor Rodrigues, Consultant Paediatric Gastroenterologist, The Children's Hospital, John Radcliffe Hospital, Oxford, UK

Laura Stewart, Community Paediatric Dietitian, Department of Nutrition and Dietetics, Royal Hospital for Sick Children, Edinburgh, UK

Sue Strudwick, Lead Clinical Specialist Speech and Language Therapist (paediatric dysphagia and complex needs), Maple Children's Centre, Kingston Hospital, Kingston, Surrey, UK

Peter B Sullivan, Reader in Paediatric Gastroenterology, Head of the Department of Paediatrics, University of Oxford, John Radcliffe Hospital, Oxford, UK

Angharad Vernon-Roberts, Clinical Research Nurse, Department of Paediatrics, University of Oxford, John Radcliffe Hospital, Oxford, UK

Foreword

It is a remarkable fact that the first two modern texts on cerebral palsy, Crothers and Paine's *The Natural History of Cerebral Palsy* (first published in 1959) and Ingram's *Paediatric Aspects of Cerebral Palsy* (first published in 1964), both do not mention feeding disorders in this population. Yet today any clinician could not fail to be aware that children with cerebral palsy may first present at 3 or 4 months with feeding difficulties, and physicians find themselves having to let the parents know that, apart from the feeding difficulties, the child has cerebral palsy. It is worth noting, too, that although this book emphasizes feeding and nutrition in cerebral palsy and other neurodevelopmental disabilities, babies with failure to thrive and, indeed, autism, will benefit from exactly the same approach as presented here.

What has led to the dramatic change in availability of information about this particular population of children? It is possibly because individuals in rather different fields – dietitians, speech and language therapists, health visitors and, indeed, paediatricians – have all found themselves seeing these children and have sought help from their colleagues in different disciplines to help them evaluate and manage the feeding problems in this population. In consequence, each discipline has learnt from the other: now nobody would set up a feeding clinic without the array of experts from different disciplines who have contributed the chapters in this book (paediatricians, speech and language therapists, nurses, dietitians), as well as other specialists such as the experienced radiologist who carries out the videofluoroscopy. All have contributed to the development of our understanding of the problems that children with neurodevelopmental disabilities often have with that most basic human need, developing the ability to self-feed.

First and foremost, however, for any feeding team are the parents, and the role that they play with their disabled child. Their role is the crucial one: they have to be confident that the advice they have been given is the right advice and also that they will be able to follow that advice. Peter Sullivan himself has studied the feelings of parents over the issues surrounding gastrostomy feeding. He is therefore able to lead a team that is very familiar with the way that parents feel, a team that is able to empathize with parents' and carers' feelings about the feeding dilemma and the need to produce an organized programme to help the child develop. They and all professionals need to be aware that often, until the child's feeding problems have been satisfactorily solved or at least attended to, further progress will not take place.

In this book, dietitians, speech and language therapists, nurses and paediatricans each report on their role. Presentation of the multidisciplinary team's approach is a basic feature of this book. There is also a specialist chapter on the gastrointestinal disorders that may require special investigation. The book ends with the growth and measurement materials that are needed by the multidisciplinary feeding team. Sullivan and his colleagues have provided us with a text that will be fundamental for anyone who has any involvement with children with neurodevelopmental disorders. It will also provide a firm basis for work with other groups of children, such as those with autism and learning difficulties, who also have depressing difficulties with feeding. Let us hope that they will see clinicians who have absorbed all they can learn from this book and will feel that they have benefited from it. Then the children and the parents will also benefit.

Martin Bax
London

Preface

The impetus to produce this book came from my colleague Dr Lewis Rosenbloom, with whom I had co-edited 'Feeding the Disabled Child' in the *Clinics in Developmental Medicine* series published by Mac Keith Press. This was in 1996, and Lewis thought that clinical practice and understanding in this field had moved on sufficiently in the intervening decade or more to warrant a further volume. I agreed on the basis that it should be written from the perspective of a multidisciplinary team actively involved in management and research in the area of feeding and nutrition in children with neurodisabilities. It should also be written by people who, as a result of their clinical contact with caregivers, would be well aware of the tremendous difficulties and problems faced by mothers (and it usually is mothers) who have to try to feed a child with significant oral motor impairment. The intention of the authors, therefore, has been to produce a work that it of practical value to health professionals both to inform them and to assist them in the care of children with neurodisabilities and their families.

I would like to express my thanks particularly to Dr Hilary Hart, Book Editor of Mac Keith Press, who has provided unfailing support, guidance and encouragement throughout all phases of the production of this book. Many clinical scientists have helped shape and inspire the views and opinions expressed in this book and it is impossible to acknowledge them all but especial thanks go to Martin Bax, Ginnie Stallings, Gordon Worley and Rich Stevenson, all of whom share the drive to improve the health and quality of life of children with neurodisabilities.

Peter B Sullivan
Oxford

Introduction

Peter B Sullivan

This book was written in response to a perceived need to present an up-to-date account of the practicalities of assessment and management of feeding problems in children with neurological impairment. The emphasis throughout the book is on multidisciplinary team working and indeed most of the contributors work together in the Feeding Clinic in the Children's Hospital, Oxford, UK. The major focus of the book is on children with cerebral palsy as these constitute the largest proportion of children with neurological impairments attending feeding clinics. Of course, there are many other neurological problems which are associated with feeding difficulties and these are listed in Box 1.1 in Chapter 1 but the principles of assessment and management are largely similar irrespective of the underlying diagnosis. Chapter 1 also presents an overview of the consequences of impairment of the neurological control of the oral motor apparatus and emphasizes that both biomedical and biopsychosocial perspectives are required for a coordinated approach to management of these problems. The second chapter from Laura Stewart (Edinburgh) and Natalie McKaig (Dundee) covers nutritional and growth assessment of neurologically impaired children with feeding difficulties and asks what we should measure, how we should make these measurements and how we should interpret what we find. Sue Strudwick in Chapter 3 then explores the impact of oral motor skills on eating and swallowing and the management strategies employed to improve these from the perspective of a specialist speech and language therapist. The approach to this topic from clinical dietitians is provided by Bridget Lambert and Wee Meng Han in Chapter 4, which in addition to detailing what is required for comprehensive dietetic assessment and management, also explores in detail the psychosocial impact of feeding problems on the caregivers of disabled children. The multidisciplinary approach to assessment and management is expanded in the chapter by Angharad Vernon-Roberts, a clinical nurse specialist who also explains what is required to support enteral nutrition by tube feeding. Tube feeding is required in those children who as a result of their neurological impairment are unable to sustain a normal nutritional state by oral feeding. Disabled children often have other consequences of neurological impairment that impact on their gastrointestinal function and which may complicate enteral tube feeding; a detailed account of these is provided in Chapter 6. Chapter 7 by Astor Rodrigues, a consultant paediatric gastroenterologist, covers the special investigations of gastrointestinal function.

A selection of real life clinical problems follows with pointers to the relevant section in the text for a more comprehensive account of the commentary provided.

Scenario 1

Billy is a 5-year-old with quadriplegic spastic cerebral palsy. He has been referred for insertion of a gastrostomy tube because of concerns about his growth. Billy cannot walk but can crawl. He has no speech and he has difficulties with chewing and swallowing but does not cough or choke and has no history of aspiration. He is exclusively orally fed with puréed and mashed food and feeding times amount to 120 minutes a day.

His weight (12 kg) and height (85 cm) are both well below the 3rd centile on standard growth charts and he has always grown at this level below and parallel to this line. His triceps skin fold thickness is 6.0 mm (15th centile).

Your advice?

1. Reassure mother and referring doctor that his nutritional state is satisfactory and that there is no need for a gastrostomy tube.
2. Arrange to insert a gastrostomy tube after excluding gastro-oesophageal reflux.
3. Advise a period of nasogastric tube feeding.
4. Add a high energy feed supplement to his existing diet.
5. Arrange a contrast videofluoroscopic examination of swallowing.

Commentary

The anthropometry on superficial analysis does not look good in that his weight is below the 3rd centile on standard growth charts, but in fact on cerebral palsy growth charts he is well within the accepted centile lines, and more importantly his triceps skin fold thickness is on the 15th centile for normal children. Samson-Fang has shown that children with cerebral palsy who have a triceps skin fold less than the 10th centile are reliably identified as those who have malnutrition.[1] So although he has oro-motor difficulties, there is no evidence that he has an unsafe swallow, and his mother is able to feed him satisfactorily without an unduly prolonged feeding time; it is arguable that she and the referring doctor can be reassured that his nutritional state is satisfactory and there is no need for a gastrostomy tube. Similarly there is no reason for providing high energy feeds or supplemental nasogastric tube feeds, and there is no evidence that he needs a videofluoroscopy as he has no history of choking or aspiration or an unsafe swallow.

See Chapter 2: Nutrition and Growth: Assessment and monitoring by Laura Stewart and Natalie A McKaig and Chapter 3: Oral Motor Impairment and Swallowing Dysfunction: Assessment and management by Sue Strudwick.

Scenario 2

Uzman was born at 24-weeks gestation and after a difficult neonatal period, now at the age of 3 years he has severe quadriplegic spastic cerebral palsy. His mother struggles to feed him as he has a tonic tongue thrust and spills most of the food offered. He also coughs and chokes during feeds and has been treated recently for pneumonia. Uzman vomits several times every day. His mother spends 4 hours each day in feeding Uzman. He has never been tube fed.

His weight (8 kg) and height (68 cm) are both well below the 3rd centile on standard growth charts and he has always grown at this level below and parallel to this line. His triceps skin fold thickness is 5.0 mm (below the 3rd centile line).

What would be your plan of management?

1. Reassure mother and referring doctor that his nutritional state is satisfactory and that there is no need for a gastrostomy tube.
2. Arrange to insert a gastrostomy tube after excluding gastro-oesophageal reflux.
3. Advise a period of nasogastric tube feeding.
4. Add a high energy feed supplement to his existing diet.
5. Arrange speech and language therapy to assist with his feeding.

Commentary

This is a boy with a severe degree of oro-motor dysfunction and an unsafe swallow, and probably gastro-oesophageal reflux, and certainly prolonged feeding time of 4 hours a day. He is underweight and has diminished energy stores as evidenced by his triceps skin fold thickness. My advice would be to arrange to insert a gastrostomy tube after excluding gastro-oesophageal reflux, and if he had this, to recommend a fundoplication at the same time. It may be necessary to institute a period of nasogastric tube feeding while these arrangements are being made, and in fact this could be advantageous, as it will be a test of whether he will tolerate tube feeding, and it wouldn't be wrong at this stage either, to offer him a high energy feed supplement to be given through the nasogastric tube.

See Chapter 6: Gastrointestinal Disorders: Assessment and management by Peter B Sullivan.

Scenario 3

Victoria is now 7 years old. She is wheelchair bound as a result of severe quadriplegic spastic cerebral palsy. When she was 3 years old gastrostomy feeding was instituted. She also had a fundoplication and does not vomit. She is fed with 1000 ml/day Paediasure Plus through the gastrostomy and now she hardly takes any food at all by mouth. Her mother says gastrostomy feeding was the best thing that was ever done for her. She has just been referred to you for follow-up because the parents have moved into your district. Her weight (30 kg) is above the 90th centile and height (110 cm) below the 10th centile on standard growth charts. Her triceps skin fold thickness is 18.0 mm (above the 90th centile line) .

Which is the most appropriate course of action?

1. Advise removal of the gastrostomy feeding tube.
2. Arrange hydrotherapy to increase her physical activity level.
3. Reduce the volume of the feed.
4. Change the feed to a low energy formula.
5. Replace the formula feed with liquidized and diluted family diet into the gastrostomy.

Commentary

This is a new patient who has been gastrostomy fed for the past 4 years, and is now clearly overweight with excessive energy stores. I suspect that her mother would not be sympathetic to removal of the gastrostomy tube. I doubt that hydrotherapy would on its own improve her body composition, although this option could be part of her overall management. Reducing the volume of the feed would probably reduce her fluid intake and therefore I would not recommend this, whereas changing the feed from a high energy 1.5 kilocalorie per kg body weight feed to a 0.75 kilocalorie per kg feed would certainly be my preferred option. I would not advise diluting the family diet into the gastrostomy because of variable nutritional content and the risk of microbial contamination.

See Chapter 4: Feeding and Dietetic Assessment and Management by Bridget Lambert and Wee Meng Han.

Scenario 4

Robyn is 10 years old she has cerebral palsy and cannot walk but she can crawl and babble and has a crude grasp. Robyn also has problematic epilepsy. Her mother spends 60 minutes each day feeding her on a mashed family diet and her nutritional state has always been considered to be satisfactory.

Six months ago feeding became a real difficulty as she started refusing oral feeds and her seizures deteriorated markedly. She lost weight significantly and a gastrostomy was inserted and this facilitated administration of her anticonvulsant medication. She is now taking an oral diet again as well as gastrostomy bolus feeds with Nutrini Multi-Fibre. She has gained weight but vomiting has emerged as a real problem (six times a day) and it has not responded to a wide range of anti-reflux medication. Lower oesophageal pH monitoring has failed on three occasions and a barium meal shows no evidence of gastro-oesophageal reflux. Histology of the oesophageal mucosa reveals mild inflammation.

Would you recommend?

1. Performance of a fundoplication.
2. Removal of the gastrostomy feeding tube.
3. Insertion of a gastrojejunostomy tube.
4. That nothing is done and that the vomiting is worth tolerating.
5. Continuous pump feeding with a whey-based formula.

Commentary

This is a difficult case in which the child's oral motor function has been good enough to maintain normal growth and nutritional state, but she has developed behavioural problems with food refusal, and it's likely that removal of the gastrostomy feeding tube would lead her to lose weight again, and provide additional problems with administration of her anti-epileptic medication. A reasonable option would be to recommend continuous pump feeding with a whey based formula to see if this stopped the vomiting.

See Chapter 4: Feeding and Dietetic Assessment and Management by Bridget Lambert and Wee Meng Han.

Scenario 5

Jake aged 6 years has cerebral palsy and after multidisciplinary assessment it is clear that he has significant oral motor dysfunction with a poor nutritional state and failure to protect his airway during swallowing. He also has forceful vomiting associated with salivation, retching, pallor and tachycardia. Lower oesophageal pH monitoring is inconclusive in terms of identifying significant gastro-oesophageal reflux (Reflux Index 9%). You are considering recommending that a gastrostomy is the best way to manage his feeding and wondering if a fundoplication is also needed.

What factors might influence your decision about this?

Commentary

It is important to realize that vomiting in children with neurological impairment is not always caused by gastro-oesophageal reflux and that activation of the emetic reflex is another important mechanism. Gastric vagal afferents are potent activators of the emetic reflex and it is possible that in some children with neurological impairment the emetic reflex is hypersensitive or there may be loss of its physiological inhibition. Such emesis is characterized by a prodrome of salivation, tachycardia, peripheral vasoconstriction, nausea and retching and, in contrast with the relatively effortless vomiting associated with gastro-oesophageal reflux, it is forceful. Vomiting accompanied by retching is seen more often in children with neurological impairment than in typical children and when this occurs preoperatively they are three times more likely to retch following fundoplication than children without retching. Retching post-fundoplication may drive the wrap at the gastro-oesophageal junction through the diaphragmatic hiatus and be associated with failure of the fundal wrap. One way forward here would be to use medical anti-emetic therapy (e.g. domperidone, ondansetron) in conjunction with a proton pump inhibitor (e.g. lansoprazole, omeprazole) rather than fundoplication following endoscopic percutaneous insertion of a gastrostomy.

See Chapter 6: Gastrointestinal Disorders: Assessment and management by Peter B Sullivan and Chapter 7: Gastrointestinal Disorders: Special investigations by Astor Rodrigues.

Scenario 6

Simon aged 3 years has had surgery to remove a brain tumour and has a residual right sided hemiplegia. He has been fed via nasogastric tube for the last 6 months; attempts by his mother and nurses to get him to eat normal food have failed as he is markedly oro-aversive.

How would you assess his ability to return to oral feeding and what management strategies would you employ to attain this goal?

Commentary

The essential elements required when weaning a child from tube feeding include:

1. promotion of a positive caregiver–child relationship;
2. a determination of the readiness of oral feeding;
3. a process of normalizing feeding; and
4. development of a behavioural feeding plan.

Determination for the readiness for oral feeding depends upon:

- an adequate nutritional status;
- a safe swallow (as judged by contrast video fluoroscopy);
- normal oral motor function; and
- caregiver readiness.

Caregiver readiness depends upon:

- the time required (weeks/months) to make this transition;
- a clear understanding of behavioural feeding techniques; and
- consistency, patience, perseverance.

Normalizing feeding is a multi-component process that involves:

1. oral stimulation (speech and language therapist input);
2. dealing with eating-related behaviour such as grimacing, mouth closure, gagging;
3. promoting an optimal feeding environment; and
4. feeding regulation by allowing hunger–satiety cues to develop and gradually decreasing tube feeds.

Before removal of the gastrostomy, one should test the ability of the child to maintain their nutritional status with oral feeding alone for a few weeks – if nutritional status is maintained then the tube can be safely removed.

See Chapter 3: Oral Motor Impairment and Swallowing Dysfunction: Assessment and management by Sue Strudwick and Chapter 5: The Multidisciplinary Team and the Practicalities of Nursing Care by Angharad Vernon-Roberts.

Reference

1. Samson-Fang LJ, Stevenson RD. Identification of malnutrition in children with cerebral palsy: poor performance of weight-for-height centiles. *Dev Med Child Neurol* 2000; **42**: 162–8.

Chapter 1

Feeding and Nutrition in Neurodevelopmental Disability: An overview

Peter B Sullivan

Introduction

The feeding and nutritional problems encountered by children with neurological impairment have been overlooked until relatively recently. Much has been written about the diagnosis and management of children with cerebral palsy and marked progress has emerged from medical and technological advances, especially with respect to mobility, communication, education and orthopaedic care.[1] Nevertheless, even as recently as the 1980s detailed accounts of the management of children with neurological impairment neglected to mention their feeding problems or the nutritional consequences of these.[2,3] It is probable that the feeding problems and growth failure were considered to be an irremediable component of these children's disorders. The central thesis in this volume is that this view is incorrect and that failure to feed and grow adequately has significant consequences for both the child and their parents and that these consequences are to a degree remediable.

The aim of this book, therefore, is to provide a framework for the multidisciplinary assessment and management of the feeding and nutritional problems in children with neurological impairment.

Oral motor impairment and swallowing dysfunction in children with neurological impairment

Oral motor impairment and swallowing dysfunction are a commonly associated disability in children with neurological impairment. Box 1.1 gives a summary of some of the more common conditions associated with oral motor impairment and swallowing dysfunction.

Box 1.1 Disorders of the central nervous system in children which may be associated with oral motor impairment and swallowing dysfunction

Acute disorders of the central nervous system

- hypoxic-ischaemic encephalopathy
- intracranial vascular events
  - infarction, haemorrhage
- infections
  - meningitis
  - encephalitis
  - poliomyelitis
- metabolic encephalopathies
  - aminoacidopathies
- trauma

Chronic – static – disorders of the central nervous system

- cerebral palsy
- genetic disorders
- Riley-Day syndrome
- kernicterus
- Arnold–Chiari malformation
- Möbius sequence

Chronic – progressive – disorders of the central nervous system

- intracranial malignancies
- degenerative conditions
  - lysosomal storage disease
  - metachromic leukodystrophy
  - adrenoleukodystrophy
  - Leigh's encephalomyelopathy
  - neuroaxonal dystrophy
  - Rett syndrome
  - Wilson's disease
  - Zellweger's disease
- multiple sclerosis
- amyotrophic lateral sclerosis
- spinal muscular atrophy
- syringobulbia

Epidemiology – cerebral palsy

Cerebral palsy is the commonest form of neurodevelopmental disability and estimates place its prevalence at 2.4 per 1000 children aged 3–10 years.[4] Recent data suggest that, contrary to initial expectations with improvements in perinatal medicine including the use of fetal monitoring and caesarean section, the prevalence of cerebral palsy has not decreased over the last 20 years.[5,6] So, although survival in babies of 24–27 completed weeks of gestation has improved, the proportion of survivors with severe disability (25%) has not changed.[7] Many survivors of neonatal intensive care will grow up with a disability so profound that they are never likely to become independently mobile, to communicate effectively with others or to feed themselves. Moreover, against this background of an unchanged prevalence of disability, there is evidence that life-expectancy is increasing in people with cerebral palsy and that this may, in part, be related to improved nutritional care in recent years.[8]

Epidemiology – feeding and nutritional problems

The literature on the incidence and prevalence of feeding difficulties mostly derives from small series reported from specialist hospital centres. More recently, robustly conducted epidemiological studies have provided an accurate measure of the extent to which children with cerebral palsy encounter feeding difficulties and have shown that this occurs in 30–40% of children sampled.[1,9] The Oxford Feeding Study, for example, in the UK examined 271 children within a defined geographical region who had cerebral palsy and feeding problems and the results (Table 1.1) convey a sense of the range of difficulties faced by these children and their caregivers.

Table 1.1 Feeding and nutritional problems in relationship to the degree of motor deficit in children with cerebral palsy (adapted from Sullivan et al, 2000)[9]

Feeding/nutritional problem	Severity of motor impairment				
	n	%	Mild	Moderate	Severe
Help with feeding needed	238/268	89	27	85	126
Choking with food	142/257	56	12	38	90
Feeding reported as stressful or not enjoyable by parent	51/262	20	5	11	35
Prolonged (≥3 hours/day) feeding times	71/258	28	3	8	60
Parents considered child underweight	93/240	38	6	25	62
Child received calorie supplements	23/271	8	1	2	20
Gastrostomy feeding	20/265	8	1	0	19
Never had feeding nutritional status assessed	169/264	64	32	77	60
Frequent vomiting	55/249	22	1	12	42
Bowels opened > every 3 days	68/267	26	5	16	47

The great majority of children with cerebral palsy , for instance, required assistance with feeding and other concerns such as frequent choking and vomiting together with prolonged feeding time contribute to mealtimes which may often be an unpleasant and frightening experience for mothers and children alike.[9]

The clear correlation between severity of feeding difficulties and the degree of motor impairment was also confirmed in the North American Growth in Cerebral Palsy Project.[1] This project was a population-based multicentre study that aimed to describe parent-reported feeding dysfunction and its association with health and nutritional status in 230 children with cerebral palsy.[1] The authors concluded that for children with moderate to severe cerebral palsy , feeding dysfunction is a common problem (occurring in around of one-third of their sample) and that it was associated with poor health (more days ill in bed, hospitalization, missed school) and poor nutritional status. The problem is not confined to those with severe oral motor dysfunction alone, even children with only mild feeding dysfunction, requiring chopped or mashed foods, may be at risk for poor nutritional status.

Another feature revealed by the Oxford Feeding Study was that there was an apparent deficit in the degree of input into feeding and nutritional issues in the care of these children. Nearly two-thirds of caregivers of these children reported that they had never had their child's feeding and nutritional state assessed. Table 1.2 (from the same study) shows that only 17% of children with cerebral palsy had contact with a dietitian in the previous 12 months. It is increasingly recognized now that early involvement of a multidisciplinary team is essential to prevent the adverse outcomes associated with feeding difficulties and poor nutritional status.[10]

Feeding and nutritional therapy are time consuming and may not be available to some children who are at greatest risk for feeding dysfunction and subsequent malnutrition.

Table 1.2 Contact of children with cerebral palsy (*n*=271) with health care professionals in the previous 12 months (adapted from Sullivan et al, 2000)[9]

Health care professional	*n*	%
Speech therapist	74	27
Occupational therapist	47	17
Dietitian	47	17
School nurse	46	17
Hospital paediatrician	55	20
Community paediatrician	33	12
Family doctor	28	10
School doctor	23	8
Health visitor	12	4
Psychologist	8	3

The lack of support – especially from paediatric dietitians – for caregivers in dealing with feeding problems was also noted in the North American study[1] which found that this may lead to significant stress in the family. This study and others have highlighted the emotional stress and adverse effect on caretaker quality of life posed by the difficulties in feeding a child with oral motor dysfunction.[1,11] High levels of psychological distress have been recorded in mothers who have a child with neurological impairment, and the greater the degree of disability in the child the greater the distress in the mother.[12] A common, and (as will be described in detail later in this book) potentially remediable, cause of this distress is prolonged feeding times related to oral motor dysfunction and inefficient feeding.

Oral motor dysfunction and its consequences

The relationship between oral motor dysfunction and growth retardation has been clearly documented.[13–15] Inefficient and slow feeding limits food intake and mothers spend prolonged periods of time (up to 8 hours a day in some cases) attempting to feed their disabled child.[16] Although prolonged feeding may compensate for feeding inefficiency when the child is small, as body size increases a point is reached at which no further compensation is possible and growth is limited by energy intake. This issue will be dealt with in detail in Chapter 3. It is important to realize, however, that oral motor dysfunction is but one of a constellation of factors – impaired communication, immobility, medication, constipation and so on (see Figure 1.1) that lead to limited food intake in children with moderate to severe cerebral palsy . Nutritional impairment from limited food intake may be further exacerbated by excess losses following vomiting and gastro-oesophageal reflux. Gastrointestinal problems are encountered in around a third of children with cerebral palsy and will be dealt with in detail in a subsequent chapter.

The outcome of limited intake when this remains untreated is undernutrition and the associated short stature, low fat stores and reduced muscle mass have been well described.[17–19]

Figure 1.2 shows anthropometric data in children with different levels of severity of cerebral palsy; severity was graded as mild (little or no difficulty walking), moderate (difficulty walking but does not need aids or a helper), and severe (needs aids and/or a helper).[17] These data reveal the significant adverse effect of cerebral palsy on linear growth and also the differential growth effect with the lower limb being more profoundly affected than the upper limb. This presumably relates to the importance of mobility and weight bearing in stimulating leg growth as the effect was significantly more marked in the group with severe motor impairment. Nevertheless, it is likely that nutritional status accounts for only 10–15% of the variability in linear growth of children with cerebral palsy.[20] It is probable that genetic and neurohumoral influences exert a greater degree of influence on linear growth than nutritional status. Wasting is, however, predominantly nutrition related and prevalent in children with severe disabilities but in the Oxford Feeding Study was also observed at an individual level in those with mild and moderate mobility defects.

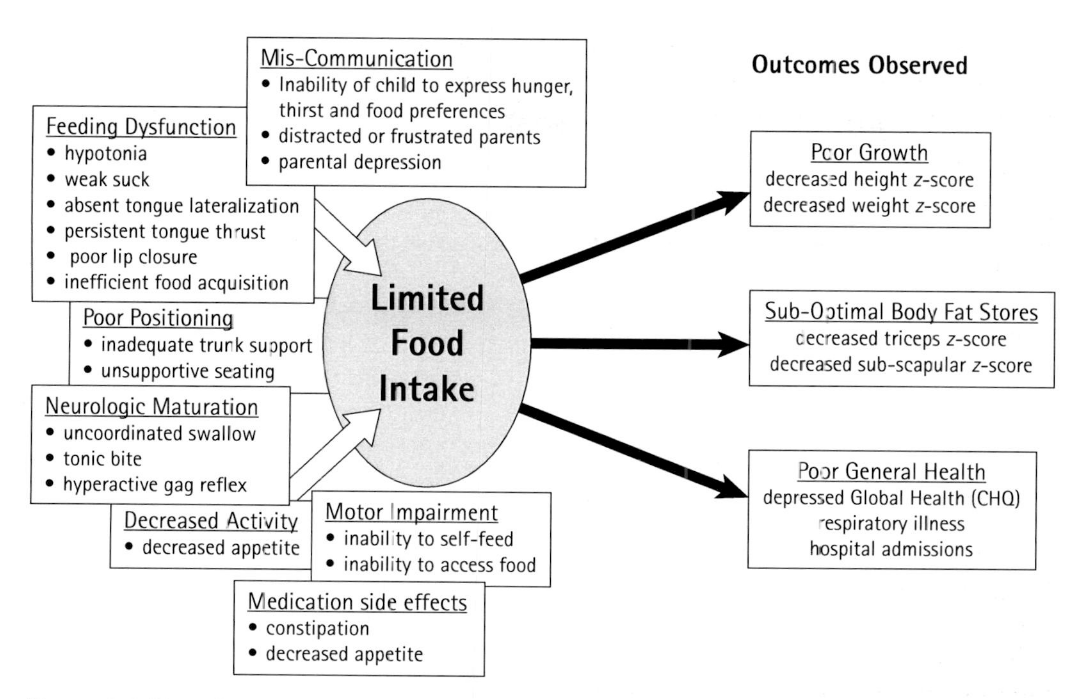

Figure 1.1 Hypothesized relationships between feeding dysfunction, motor impairment, communication and growth, and health status outcomes in children with moderate to severe cerebral palsy. Reproduced from the Journal of the American Dietetic Association, Vol 102(3), 361–373. Fung EB, Samson-Fang L, Stallings VA, Conaway M, Liptak G, Henderson RC, Worley G, O'Donnell M, Calvert R, Rosenbaum P, Chumlea W, Stevenson RD. Feeding dysfunction is associated with poor growth and health status in children with cerebral palsy. With permission from Elsevier. CHQ, child health questionnaire.

Problems with reference standards

The body composition of the child with severe cerebral palsy differs from that of the average child; a decrease in body cell mass accompanies an expansion of the extracellular fluid volume. The relative immobility of the child with severe cerebral palsy reduces fat free mass (largely muscle but also skeletal mass) as well as energy expenditure. The reduced energy expenditure of children with cerebral palsy is reflected in a lower dietary energy requirement – around 80% of current recommendations for children without neurological impairment. These differences in body composition and energy expenditure, therefore, mean that standard reference data for ideal nutritional input and optimal growth do not apply to children with cerebral palsy. This is a problem for those involved in the nutritional care of children with cerebral palsy because growth assessment requires reliable measures and comparison reference data. Only recently has an attempt been made to produce growth charts derived from observations made on clearly defined samples of children with cerebral palsy and which have been stratified by level of motor functioning and feeding ability.[19,21] Appendix 1

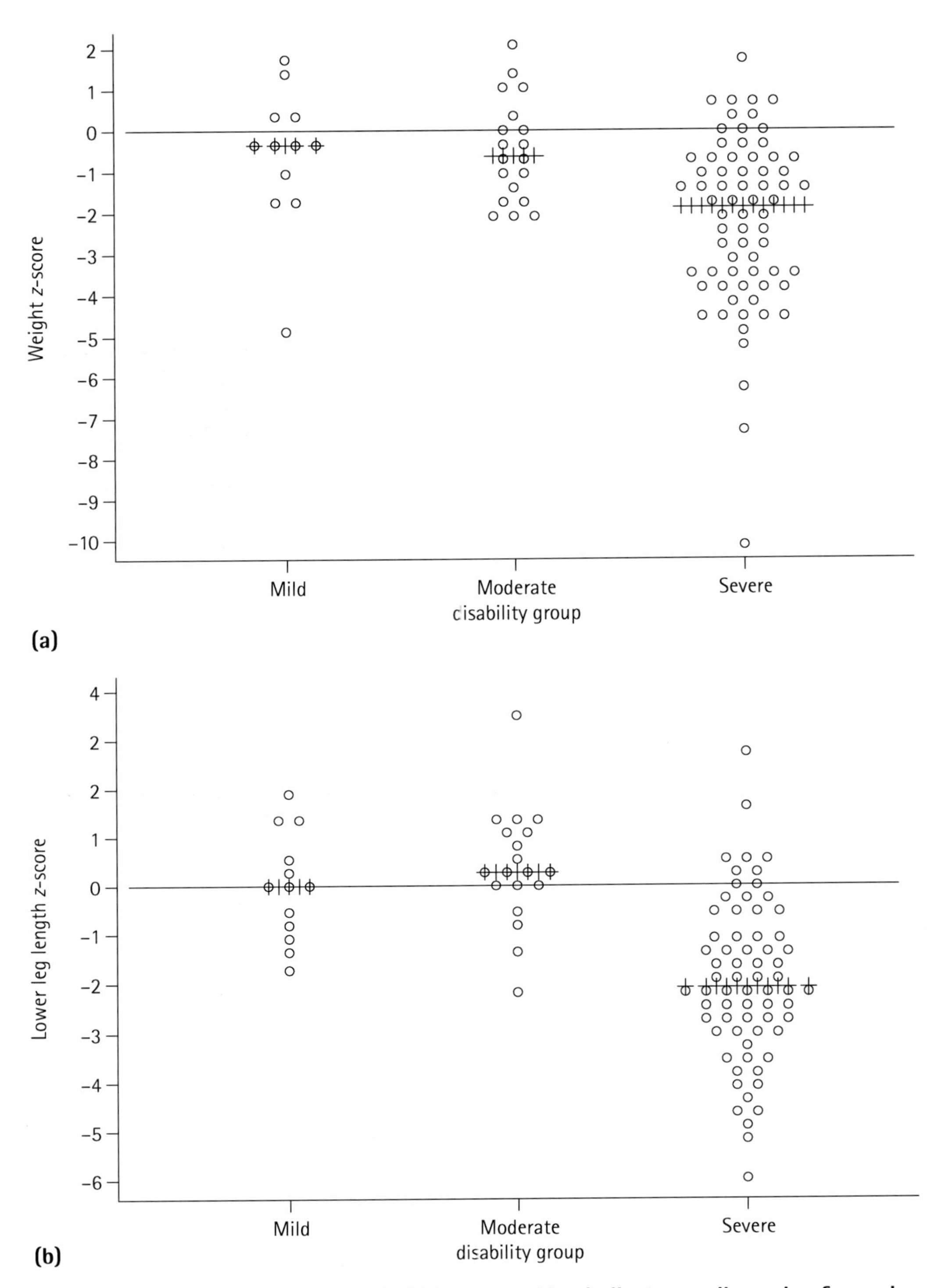

Figure 1.2 Dotplot of *z*-scores by disability group. Line indicates median value for each disability group (a) bodyweight; (b) lower leg length

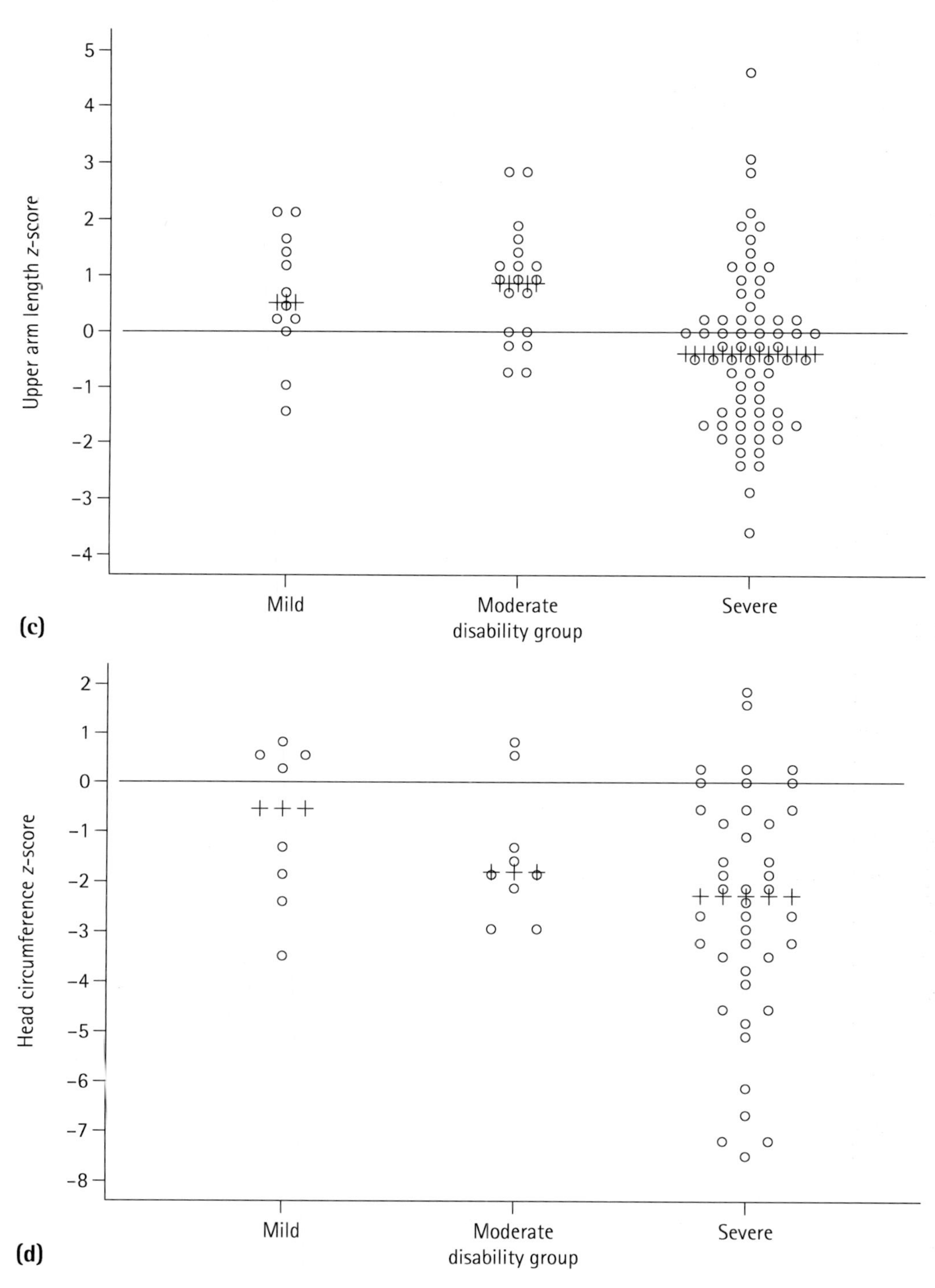

Figure 1.2 Dotplot of *z*-scores by disability group. Line indicates median value for each disability group (c) upper arm length; (d) head circumference *z*-score by disability group.

contains a series of growth charts for children with different levels of motor disability and for those who are also fed by gastrostomy tube. It is important to note, however, that these are *descriptive* in nature, i.e. they reveal how children with different levels of motor impairment actually grow – but they are not 'reference standards'.

Nevertheless, the advent of these growth charts is welcome as the poor performance of standard reference charts in identifying malnourished cerebral palsy children has been recognized for a long time. Samson-Fang and Stevenson (2000), for instance, have shown that a triceps skin fold thickness (TSF) performs much more accurately than weight-for-height in identifying those with depleted fat stores and that a TSF below the 10th centile identifies 96% of malnourished children with cerebral palsy.[22]

Once malnutrition is identified the next problem is to decide how much to feed the child. The central consideration here is the amount of energy that the child requires to grow optimally. There is a wide variation in total energy expenditure (largely attributable to variations in physical activity levels) in immobile children with cerebral palsy. This individual variation, together with the lack of any suitable reference standards, compounds the difficulties in writing an accurate dietetic prescription. Fortunately there are some common sense 'rules of thumb' derived from experimental and clinical observations that can guide the clinical management of children with cerebral palsy. For instance, as the energy requirement for growth relative to maintenance is small (about 10 kj/g), satisfactory growth can be used as a sensitive indicator of whether energy needs are being met. It is surprising how little may be required to achieve this. Thus, exclusively gastrostomy-tube fed children with cerebral palsy grow consistently on an energy intake of less than 7 kcal/cm i.e. diets ranging from 500–1100 kcal/day which is 16–50% less than the recommended daily allowance.[23] Such extremely low energy intakes often make paediatricians, nurses and dietitians hesitant to accept the adequacy of these diets. The consequences of this particularly in the gastrostomy fed child with cerebral palsy may be overfeeding and the risk of excessive fat storage.[24]

Treatment of suboptimal nutrition

Undernutrition has significant consequences for the child with cerebral palsy . There is hardly any physiological function which is not compromised by poor nutrition. Some examples of these will be described. Skeletal muscles are weakened further, which for the respiratory system renders the cough weak and predisposes the child (already at risk from aspiration secondary to oral motor dysfunction) to respiratory infection. The risk of infection is further increased as proper functioning of the immune system is compromised by undernutrition. Cardiac output is reduced and circulation time prolonged (Figure 1.3).

When the nutritional problems caused by feeding difficulty are properly addressed the consequences of undernutrition for the child are revealed. One of the first signs reported by parents is that the cold, pale and mottled condition of arms and legs (Figure 1.3) disappears as the limbs become pink and warm.[25] Weight gain in the child is also

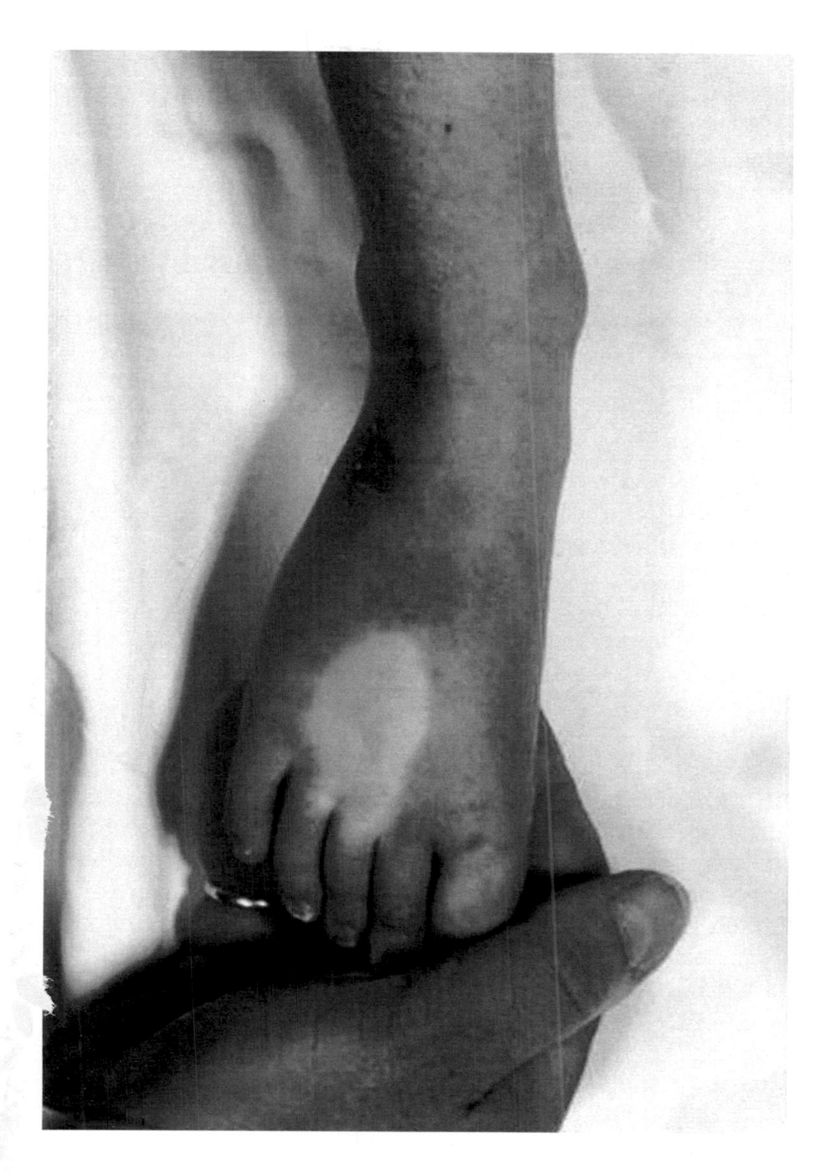

Figure 1.3
Poor peripheral circulation in an undernourished child with cerebral palsy. Note also the slow healing skin abrasion on the dorsal aspect of the foot.

associated with an improvement in overall health and reduction in hospital attendances and frequency of chest infections have been reported following nutritional restitution.[26]

Adequate nutrition is also associated with an improvement in levels of alertness and mood and parents report that the child is 'brighter'. Some published reports have noted significant developmental progress in previously undernourished children with cerebral palsy accompanying improved nutritional status.[27] This effect of nutrition on neurodevelopmental status is a feature that remains to be fully explored especially when children at risk are identified early and adequate nutritional management instituted before the onset of malnutrition.

Psychosocial considerations

The central thesis in this volume is that nutritional compromise from failure to feed adequately has significant consequences and is to a degree remediable and it has been approached largely from the standpoint of a biomedical model of health. There is a growing body of qualitative research which points to the need to incorporate a 'biopsychosocial' component to health care especially when interacting with the parents of children with neurological impairment.[16,28] Medical emphasis on growth and health may overlook parental concerns about oral and tube feeding. Mothers, who may harbour feelings of guilt about their child's poor growth, can perceive the suggestion that gastrostomy feeding is required as confirmation of failure. Fears about loss of normal eating, dependency on gastrostomy feeds, complications of the procedure and so on can make parents very resistant to the idea of supplemental tube feeding and even if they agree they may opt to use the tube only as a last resort. Thus, a great deal of sensitivity to the fears and feelings of the parents is required when approaching the subject of gastrostomy tube feeding. Furthermore, all members within the multidisciplinary team should be well informed about the indications for and advantages and disadvantages of tube feeding so that a consistent message is conveyed to parents. In the experience of the author there is no better way to assist parents with the decision about whether or not to proceed with gastrostomy in their disabled child when it is clearly indicated than by introducing them to others in a similar situation that have experience of this intervention.

Recurrent pain and irritability

Another issue of great concern to caregivers is the occurrence in their disabled child of persistent irritability often ascribed to chronic or recurrent pain. Given that it is difficult to obtain reliable measures of the degree of pain or a clear indication of the source of pain in a child with a communication disorder, it is perhaps not surprising that this problem has not received much attention in the literature. This issue is covered here because such studies as have been undertaken point to the gastrointestinal tract as a commonly suspected source of recurrent pain. In one study, for instance, more than a third of children with severe cognitive impairment experienced pain that lasted for hours each week and the gastrointestinal tract was the commonest non-accidental source of pain.[29] Results from the North American Growth in Cerebral Palsy project suggest that around 10% of caregivers report that their children experience pain on a regular basis.[30] This study also demonstrated that pain was related to the severity of motor impairment and the presence of a gastrostomy feeding tube and taking medications for gastrointestinal symptoms (e.g. gastro-oesophageal reflux (GOR), motility problems and constipation). Manometric studies have shown that upper gastrointestinal sensory disorders contribute not only to abdominal discomfort in children with cerebral palsy but also to persistent feeding problems in these children.[31] Visceral hyperalgesia may result from a range of sensitizing gastrointestinal disorders including GOR, fundoplication, gastrostomy insertion, chronic constipation coupled with the disordered cross-talk between the cerebral cortex and the enteric nervous system that occurs in children with cerebral palsy. A range of pharmacological approaches to modulate neurotransmission in the enteric nervous system (e.g.

imipramine, amitryptyline, cyproheptadine) or to inhibit central sensitization (e.g. gabapentin) have been shown to have therapeutic value.[31,32]

References

1. Fung EB, Samson-Fang L, Stallings VA et al. Feeding dysfunction is associated with poor growth and health status in children with cerebral palsy. *J Am Diet Assoc* 2002; **102**: 3–73.
2. Evans P, Elliott M, Alberman E, Evans S. Prevalence and disabilities in 4 to 8 year olds with cerebral palsy. *Arch Dis Child* 1985; **60**: 940–5.
3. Vining EP, Accardo PJ, Rubenstein JE, Farrell SE, Roizen NJ. Cerebral palsy. A pediatric developmentalist's overview. *Am J Dis Child* 1976; **130**: 643–9.
4. Boyle CA, Yeargin-Allsopp M, Doernberg NS, Holmgreen P, Murphy CC, Schendel DE. Prevalence of selected developmental disabilities in children 3–10 years of age: the Metropolitan Atlanta Developmental Disabilities Surveillance Program, 1991. *MMWR CDC Surveill* 1996; **45**: 1–14.
5. Winter S, Autry A, Boyle C, Yeargin-Allsopp M. Trends in the prevalence of cerebral palsy in a population-based study. *Pediatrics* 2002; **110**: 1220–5.
6. Horbar JD, Badger GJ, Carpenter JH et al. Trends in mortality and morbidity for very low birth weight infants, 1991–1999. *Pediatrics* 2002; **110**: 143–51.
7. Wood NS, Costeloe K, Gibson AT, Hennessy EM, Marlow N, Wilkinson AR. The EPICure study: associations and antecedents of neurological and developmental disability at 30 months of age following extremely preterm birth. *Arch Dis Child Fetal Neonatal Ed* 2005; **90**: F134–40.
8. Strauss D, Shavelle R, Reynolds R, Rosenbloom L, Day S. Survival in cerebral palsy in the last 20 years: signs of improvement? *Dev Med Child Neurol* 2007; **49**: 86–92.
9. Sullivan PB, Lambert B, Rose M, Ford-Adams M, Johnson A, Griffiths P. Prevalence and severity of feeding and nutritional problems in children with neurological impairment: Oxford Feeding Study. *Dev Med Child Neurol* 2000; **42**: 10–80.
10. Marchand V, Motil KJ. Nutrition support for neurologically impaired children: a clinical report of the North American Society for Pediatric Gastroenterology, Hepatology, and Nutrition. *J Pediatr Gastroenterol Nutr* 2006; **43**: 123–35.
11. Sullivan PB, Juszczak E, Bachlet AM et al. Impact of gastrostomy tube feeding on the quality of life of carers of children with cerebral palsy. *Dev Med Child Neurol* 2004; **46**: 796–800.
12. Sloper P, Turner S. Risk and resistance factors in the adaptation of parents of children with severe physical disability. *J Child Psychol Psychiatry* 1993; **34**: 167–88.
13. Krick J, Van Duyn MA. The relationship between oral-motor involvement and growth: a pilot study in a pediatric population with cerebral palsy. *J Am Diet Assoc* 1984; **84**: 555–9.
14. Gisel EG, Applegate-Ferrante T, Benson JE, Bosma JF. Effect of oral sensorimotor treatment on measures of growth, eating efficiency and aspiration in the dysphagic child with cerebral palsy. *Dev Med Child Neurol* 1995; **37**: 528–43.
15. Dahl M, Thommessen M, Rasmussen M, Selberg T. Feeding and nutritional characteristics in children with moderate or severe cerebral palsy. *Acta Paediatr* 1996; **85**: 697–701.
16. Craig GM, Scambler G, Spitz L. Why parents of children with neurodevelopmental disabilities requiring gastrostomy feeding need more support. *Dev Med Child Neurol* 2003; **45**: 183–8.
17. Sullivan PB, Juszczak E, Lambert BR, Rose M, Ford-Adams ME, Johnson A. Impact of feeding problems on nutritional intake and growth: Oxford Feeding Study II. *Dev Med Child Neurol* 2002; **44**: 461–7.
18. Samson-Fang L, Fung E, Stallings VA et al. Relationship of nutritional status to health and societal participation in children with cerebral palsy. *J Pediatr* 2002; **141**: 637–43.
19. Stevenson RD, Conaway M, Chumlea WC et al. Growth and health in children with moderate-to-severe cerebral palsy. *Pediatrics* 2006; **118**: 1010–18.

20. Stallings VA, Charney EB, Davies JC, Cronk CE. Nutrition-related growth failure of children with quadriplegic cerebral palsy. *Dev Med Child Neurol* 1993; **35**: 126–38.
21. Krick J, Murphy-Miller P, Zeger S, Wright E. Pattern of growth in children with cerebral palsy. *J Am Diet Assoc* 1996; **96**: 680–5.
22. Samson-Fang LJ, Stevenson RD. Identification of malnutrition in children with cerebral palsy: poor performance of weight-for-height centiles. *Dev Med Child Neurol* 2000; **42**: 162–8.
23. Bandini LG, Puelzl-Quinn H, Morelli JA, Fukagawa NK. Estimation of energy requirements in persons with severe central nervous system impairment. *J Pediatr* 1995; **126**: 828–32.
24. Sullivan PB, Alder N, Bachlet AM et al. Gastrostomy feeding in cerebral palsy: too much of a good thing? *Dev Med Child Neurol* 2006; **48**: 877–82.
25. Patrick J, Boland M, Stoski D, Murray GE. Rapid correction of wasting in children with cerebral palsy. *Dev Med Child Neurol* 1986; **28**: 734–9.
26. Sullivan PB, Morrice JS, Vernon-Roberts A, Grant H, Eltumi M, Thomas AG. Does gastrostomy tube feeding in children with cerebral palsy increase the risk of respiratory morbidity? *Arch Dis Child* 2006; **91**: 478–82.
27. Sanders KD, Cox K, Cannon R et al. Growth response to enteral feeding by children with cerebral palsy. *J Parenter Enteral Nutr* 1990; **14**: 23–6.
28. Sleigh G. Mothers' voice: a qualitative study on feeding children with cerebral palsy. *Child Care Health Dev* 2005; **31**: 373–83.
29. Breau LM, Camfield CS, McGrath PJ, Finley GA. The incidence of pain in children with severe cognitive impairments. *Arch Pediatr Adolesc Med* 2003; **157**: 1219–26.
30. Houlihan CM, O'Donnell M, Conaway M, Stevenson RD. Bodily pain and health-related quality of life in children with cerebral palsy. *Dev Med Child Neurol* 2004; **46**: 305–10.
31. Zangen T, Ciarla C, Zangen S, et al. Gastrointestinal motility and sensory abnormalities may contribute to food refusal in medically fragile toddlers. *J Pediatr Gastroenterol Nutr* 2003; **37**: 287–93.
32. Hauer JM, Wical BS, Charnas L. Gabapentin successfully manages chronic unexplained irritability in children with severe neurologic impairment. *Pediatrics* 2007; **119**: e519–22.

Chapter 2

Nutrition and Growth: Assessment and monitoring

Laura Stewart and Natalie A McKaig

Introduction

This chapter is concerned with children with neurological impairment who have been referred to a team or health professional because of concerns that they may have faltering growth and/or have a poor nutritional status. The term neurological impairment is used throughout but readers should note that most of the work carried out in this area has been undertaken in children with cerebral palsy. Although the authors believe that the overall principles discussed are relevant to other children with neurodevelopmental disability, caution is needed when extrapolating to other neurological conditions. Different health professionals may use different definitions of faltering growth and failure to thrive and use the terms interchangeably; we have used the common practice definition of faltering growth to mean when a child's weight or height remains constant over time thus appearing on the growth charts as a horizontal line and the more urgent scenario where the weight has fallen down crossing through two centile lines of the growth chart.

It is important that the initial assessment and subsequent monitoring of these children is done in as systematic manner as possible. A multidisciplinary team approach to assessing and monitoring children with neurological impairment and faltering growth is the most suitable and successful. In this chapter we will discuss the appropriate methods for health professionals to use in the initial nutritional assessment and subsequent nutritional monitoring of such children. These procedures may be carried out by one or more members of the multidisciplinary team and will depend on the make up of each local team.

Frequently asked questions by dietitians and other professionals include the following.

- What should we be measuring in these children?
- How should we be making these measurements?

- How often should we measure them?
- What dietary assessments should we be doing?
- What are the ideal nutritional indicators and biochemical markers?

This chapter is based on our systematic review of the literature[1,2] and current best practice; however, it should be noted that at this time the evidence base remains uncertain.

Initial assessment

When a child is referred to a health professional or a team because of concerns over possible faltering growth or poor nutritional intake, it is important that a well-conducted assessment is carried out. This should include reviewing their:

- present weight and height (or proxy);
- previous growth history;
- eating and drinking ability;
- relevant biochemical and haematological indices.

All of these are discussed in detail below.

Measurements

Weight

A child's growth should be dynamic and therefore a series of weight and height measurements that have been taken sequentially are required. The health professional must obtain an accurate weight history either from the parent held records, hospital medical, community child health or school nursing records.

Measuring weight for children with neurological impairment can be difficult and Stevenson recommends measuring on the most appropriate weighing equipment for the individual child and situation.[2] There are several methods of weighing that are commonly used for children with neurological impairment: wheelchair scales, sitting and hoist scales. Weighing is often carried out with the carer holding the child on either sitting or standing scales then subtracting the carer's weight. The exact method used is usually dependent on local circumstances. Interestingly no studies comparing the different methods have been carried out to date. For follow up monitoring (see below) and accurate comparison of serial measurements, the same scales and method should be used each time. Ideally, the same person should carry out the measurements to reduce the chances of error and ensure consistency but this is not always possible. This last point highlights the need for proper regular training in anthropometric techniques for all staff concerned.

Weight measurements should be plotted on gender specific growth centile charts to ascertain if the child is following an appropriate curve. Great care needs to be taken when interpreting standard growth charts when used for children with neurological impairment (see below). Recently descriptive growth charts specific for use in children with different levels of motor impairment secondary to cerebral palsy have become available (see Appendix 1).

Height

Height measurements should also be taken sequentially and plotted on growth charts; however, for many children with neurological impairment this is the most difficult measurement to obtain. When a child can stand, height measured using a stadiometer is the ideal method. Supine length is a good alternative provided it can be assured that the child's posture and limb alignment are lying straight. When neither is possible or it is likely to be inaccurate e.g. if limb contractures, scoliosis or kyphosis are present, then an alternative height measurement is necessary.[2–6] A short description of these alternative techniques is given below and illustrated in Figures 2.1–2.4.

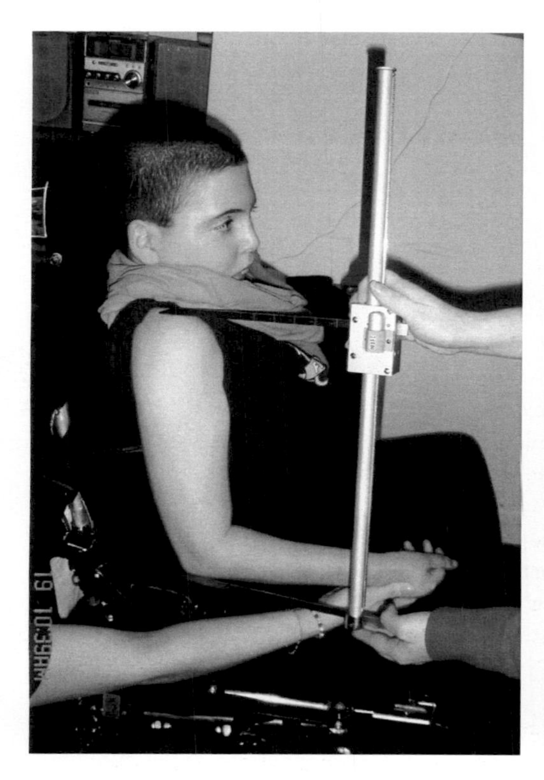

Figure 2.1 Measurement of upper arm length using anthropometer.

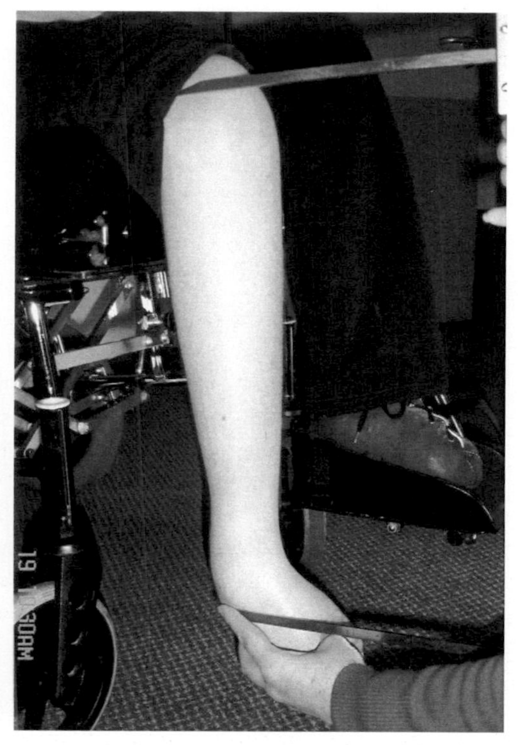

Figure 2.2 Measurement of lower leg length (tibial length) using anthropometer.

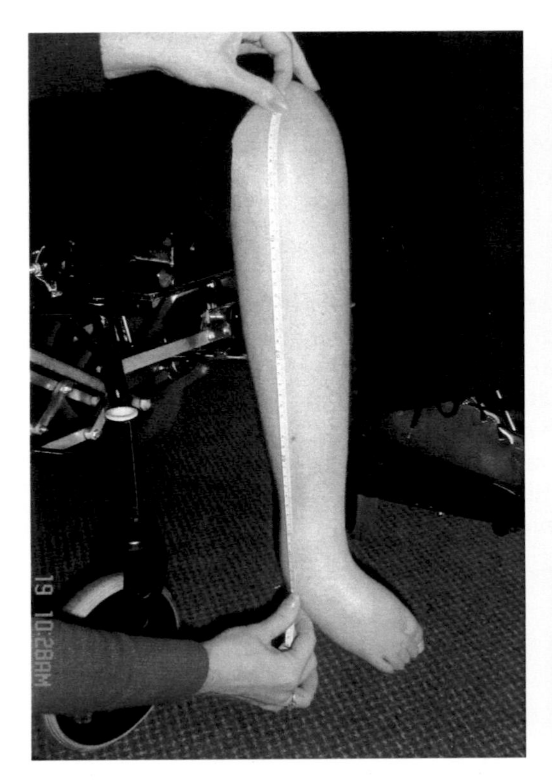

Figure 2.3 Measurement of lower leg length (tibial length) using a steel tape measure.

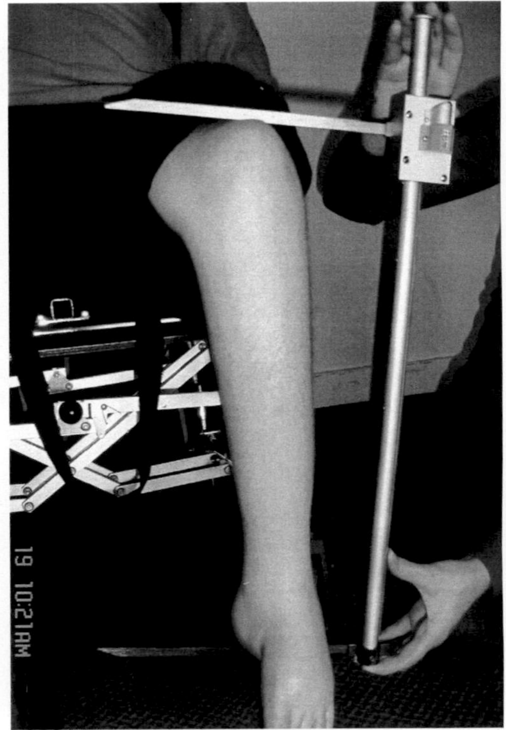

Figure 2.4 Measurement of knee height using anthropometer.

Box 2.1 Alternative height measurements[7]

Upper arm length is measured from the acromion to the head of the radius; it should be taken on the right side or the least affected side. Two measurements are taken and then averaged. It can only be taken accurately using an anthropometer.[8]

The lower leg length (also know as the tibial length) is measured from the top of the tibia to the distal tip of the medial malleolus (sphyron). It requires the child to be sitting and is taken on the right side or the least affected side. This measurement can be taken accurately with an anthropometer or with a steel measuring tape. Two measurements are taken and averaged.[9]

Knee height is measured with the child sitting down and the knee and ankle bent to 90°. Using a sliding calliper the distance between the heel to the anterior surface of the thigh over the femoral condyle is measured, on the left side or least affected side. Two measurements are taken and averaged.[9]

Weight and height should be monitored (see below) using the same tool and method every time to allow an accurate comparison to be made.

Growth charts
To date it is usual practice to plot the weights and heights of children with neurological impairment using the standard centile growth charts (either Child Growth Foundation[a] or Castlemead[b] in the UK and www.cdc.gov/growthcharts/ in the USA). It is important to note when interpreting the weight and height growth charts in this client group that many children's measurements may lie below the 0.4th centile on the Child Growth Foundation charts or the 3rd centile of the Castlemead growth charts. Although the pattern of 'normal' growth for disabled children is still unclear, it is common practice to view appropriate growth as plotted weights and heights over time following the general curve of the centile lines. At the same time both weight and height curves should be in proportion to each other. Interestingly in a study attempting to develop specific growth charts for children with cerebral palsy, Krick et al found that the 50th centile for both weight and height for children with cerebral palsy was below the 10th centile on the US NHANES standard growth charts.[8] Recently growth charts specific for use in children with different levels of motor impairment secondary to cerebral palsy have become available (see Appendix 1).

Body mass index
At present there is no evidence in the literature supporting the use of body mass index (BMI) in this client group. Indeed one study found BMI to be a poor indicator of low body fat in children with cerebral palsy.[9] In clinical practice in children with neurological impairment BMI is not always a useful tool, as in children with both poor weight gain and stunted height growth a calculated BMI may appear 'acceptable' when plotted on centile charts.

It should be noted that the use of BMI in children with neurological impairment who are *overweight or obese* is entirely appropriate.

Anthropometric arm measurements
Skin fold thickness can be measured at various sites in the body using measurement callipers and are a proxy for estimating body fat. The measurements should be painless but do require to be undertaken by a trained person. The most common sites for taking measurements are at the triceps, the suprailiac crest and the subscapula. Mid-arm (also known as upper mid-arm) circumference is a measurement taken at the midpoint of the upper arm using a measuring tape. The mid-arm circumference and the skin fold thickness measurements can then be inserted in an equation to estimate

a Child Growth Foundation growth charts available form Harlow Printing Ltd, Maxwell Street, South Shields, Tyne & Wear, NE33 4PU.

b Castlemead Publications, Swains Mill, 4A Crane Mead, Ware, Herts, SG12 9PY.

body fat and lean body mass. There are standard centiles for all these measurements for comparison.

There is good support in the literature for the use of tricep skin fold thickness, mid-arm circumference and mid-arm muscle circumference, as estimations of body fat and muscle in this patient group.[2,4,9] Samson-Fang and Stevenson in 2000 showed that a tricep skin fold thickness measurement below the 10th centile was a good indicator of low body fat stores in children with cerebral palsy.[9]

Measurements can either be directly compared with tables produced by Frisancho[10] or plotted on centile charts available from Castlemead Publications (see above). Again health professionals should be aware when interpreting these centile charts that they are based on work with children without neurological impairments.

In routine practice it can be difficult to take accurate skin fold thickness measurements in some children with neurological impairment. The subscapular skin fold thickness measurement can be impractical in day to day practice because of the need to remove clothing and/or spinal jackets. By contrast the triceps skin fold thickness is much easier to perform in the clinical setting and provides a reliable indication of a child's nutritional and energy balance status.[9] We would recommend that health professionals should not undertake these measurements unless they have had training in the techniques. As for other measurements, the same person should, ideally, perform all measurements on an ongoing basis.

Dietary and feeding assessment

It is important to be aware that there are many organic and non-organic reasons why children with neurological impairment may exhibit growth faltering. On the whole these can be related to their difficulty or inability to take in sufficient energy for growth or even to maintain weight. A child's feeding ability has been shown to be directly associated with their nutritional status.[11]

Possible causes of inadequate nutritional intake include:

- poor self-feeding ability and a reliance on others for all their nutritional intake;
- inability to express hunger or thirst;
- poor sucking, swallowing or chewing abilities;
- gastro-oesophageal reflux, vomiting or aspiration;
- texture modification such as liquidizing or mashing of food which can lead to a diluting of the nutrients and energy content of the food;
- behavioural problems particularly around food and mealtimes;
- inappropriate intake for age e.g. school-aged children taking baby food or milk from a bottle with a teat; although the texture may be appropriate the nutritional content is inadequate.

This is a complex issue and we recommend that dietary assessments and estimations of nutritional intakes should only be carried out by an experienced paediatric dietitian. Dietary assessments are an important tool for dietitians; there are three commonly used methods of dietary assessment: food records; recall; and food frequency questionnaires. A number of studies emphasize that these methods give inaccurate estimations of nutritional intakes in this patient group.[2,12] Stallings et al found that the energy intakes of a group of children with cerebral palsy were over-reported by 44–54% more than their actual energy intake.[13] Therefore dietary assessments alone are unlikely to be useful and, if employed, should be interpreted with caution. Observing a meal may be especially helpful in enabling the dietitian to see the actual volume and types of food and drink offered and taken by a child as well as viewing all factors that affect dietary intake such as posture and environment.[12] It is especially informative to observe the feeding routine in the home environment; although a home visit is ideal it may not be practical but a video recording provided by the parent/carer is a useful substitute for this.

Several studies have highlighted the importance of a simple feeding assessment in recognizing children 'at risk' of under nutrition.[12,14,15] These studies indicated that an assessment of a child's feeding competence, using a basic scoring system, by a speech and language therapist provides vital information for identifying children at risk from poor nutritional status. Assessment of the safety of the swallow is also important when determining an intervention plan. Therefore a full eating and swallowing assessment conducted by an appropriately trained speech and language therapist will give the team a perspective on the holistic picture of the child's eating and drinking ability. This is an area where paediatric dietitians and speech and language therapists work closely together, particularly when giving advice to parents and carers about appropriate consistency and nutrient density of foods. This area is discussed in-depth in Chapter 3.

Biochemical and haematological indices

Biochemical and haematological indices may be useful in identifying nutritional inadequacies or abnormalities such as iron deficiency anaemia, high vitamin A or low selenium levels. This is of particular importance in monitoring children on home enteral tube feeding (HETF); however, there is no consensus on the appropriate indices to be monitored in these children. The Parental and Enteral Nutrition Group of the British Dietetic Association have made recommendations for monitoring adults on HETF.[16] It seems prudent to follow best practice for biochemical and haematological indices to be measured in children: Box 2.2 is based on recommendations by NHS Lothian, Scotland, UK.[17] It is recommended that these measurements are taken at baseline and then at least once a year. This, however, should be considered as best practice and has not been fully evaluated. This is an area for further research and clarification.

Box 2.2 Recommended biochemical and haematological indices

- Urea and electrolytes
- Creatinine
- Glucose
- Liver function tests
- Calcium/phosphate/magnesium
- Albumin/protein
- Full blood count
- Haemoglobin
- Zinc, copper, selenium
- Vitamins A/D/E/B_{12}
- Parahormone
- Folate
- Ferritin

Estimating nutrient requirements

A recent systemic review of the literature has shown that there is no good quality evidence to enable health professionals to calculate or estimate the appropriate energy, protein, fluid, vitamins and minerals for children with cerebral palsy (unpublished work). There does, however, appear to be evidence that the majority of these children do not have the same nutritional requirements as children without neurological impairment. Sullivan et al concluded that 80% of children with cerebral palsy consumed a diet that was lower in energy than that of children without disability. They also suggested that nutrient reference ranges for mainstream healthy children may be inappropriate for this client group.[11] Thomas and Akobeng highlighted that even when energy intake is adequate micronutrient intake may not be, resulting in multiple nutritional deficiencies.[18]

Energy, protein and nutrient requirements for this client group may be below those cited in the Department of Health's Dietary Reference Values book.[19] Energy requirements need to be estimated on an individual basis taking into account the child's current weight, previous growth, estimated present energy intake and feeding ability. Health professionals must be aware that some children with neurological impairment when tube fed can become obese and that close monitoring of rate of weight gain is essential, particularly when initiating tube feeding (see below). In practice protein, vitamins and minerals intakes that fall between the reference nutritional intakes (RNI) and lower reference nutritional intakes (LRNI) for age, weight age or height age are usually taken as being acceptable.[20]

Fluid intake is also an essential aspect of the nutritional intake of these children and should always be considered. In routine practice fluid requirements for children are estimated using the tables and calculations in the Great Ormond Street Hospital's booklet on nutritional requirements for children in health and disease.[20] Great caution should be shown, however, when using these tables for estimating the fluid requirements for children with neurological impairment; for a significant number of children, particularly those who are enterally fed, there is a problem with toleration of volume of fluid which can lead to vomiting when inappropriate large volumes of fluid are given at one time or over 24 hours. If children are passing adequate volumes of urine which is not dark or does not have a strong odour then this is a good indication that the child is receiving adequate volumes of fluid.

Planning nutritional intervention

Once a child is considered to exhibit faltering growth there are a number of options for improving nutritional intake. Increasing the energy density of food is of vital importance to reverse weight loss or poor weight gain; however, protein and the other micronutrients (nutrient density) as discussed above should always be considered.

There are three levels of dietary intervention that should be considered in this client group:

- increasing portion sizes;
- use of special dietary supplement;
- enteral tube feeding.

The first, increasing portion sizes and giving more of favourite foods, is the simplest and for some children can be effective. Parents and carers should also be encouraged to use high energy foods such as full fat milk and creamy yoghurts: see the list of high energy foods in Box 2.3. Small portions (of high energy foods) should be offered frequently throughout the day e.g. offer two courses at lunch and tea with snacks mid-morning and mid-afternoon and at supper.

Box 2.3 High energy foods

Consider the following:

- add more butter, grated cheese to food e.g. mashed potatoes;
- use energy dense foods
- use thick sauces e.g. white sauce to moisten food;
- use thick and creamy yoghurts;
- add cream, evaporated milk to puddings;
- add cream to soup, dilute condensed soup with milk;
- add cooked meat to soup;
- use full fat dairy products.

The second option is the use of special dietary products (also known as borderline substances as they can be prescribed for certain medically defined conditions) that are available to the children on NHS prescription. There are a number of products either in powder or liquid forms: carbohydrate sources, fat sources or a mixture of carbohydrate and fat that can be added to food and drinks to optimize energy intake. These products are often very useful in this group, as the children are generally not asked to take extra volume of food or drinks. Supplementary drinks that can be milk or fruit or yoghurt based and come in small cartons are frequently used. These tend to contain 1 kcal or 1.5 kcal per ml as well as protein, vitamins and minerals. High protein/high energy puddings are also available on prescription. The nutrient intake of these supplements should not exceed safe nutrient intakes for height age/age e.g. vitamin A.

For a number of children who cannot take in adequate nutrition orally or who have an unsafe swallow, home enteral tube feeding (HETF) will be used. Indeed according to the British Artificial Nutrition Survey (BANS) database disabled children make up the largest proportion of children using HETF in the UK.[20] There will be some children for whom enteral nutrition is their sole source of nutrition and others where it is supplementary to their oral diet. Enteral tube feeding is discussed in Chapters 5–7.

It is very important to note that if there is a safe swallow oral food should be offered at every mealtime even if only small amounts are taken and a supplementary tube feed is required. Oral feeding should not continue if there is an unsafe swallow (assessed by a speech and language therapist and preferably in conjunction with videofluoroscopic imaging – see Chapters 4 and 6) or the experience is unpleasant/traumatic for the child.

Supplementary tube feeding may initially be quite difficult for parents/carers to accept but it can eventually help reduce stress at mealtimes and leave more time for other social activities. Tube feeding should, where possible, be discussed with parents/carers as early as possible and the advantages and disadvantages discussed to enable an informed decision to be made. A multidisciplinary team approach is of paramount importance in such situations so that conflicting advice is not given and the family feel supported. It is vital that any tube feeding regime fits into the child's and family daily routine rather than expecting their lifestyle to fit into a feeding regime.

Follow up monitoring

Continuous nutritional monitoring of children who have been commenced on nutritional supplements or HETF is essential to ensure that they are growing appropriately and remain on the most suitable feeding regime for age and optimal growth. The frequency of monitoring will be determined to some extent by local circumstances and policy. Our review of the literature found only one report that recommended the frequency of measurements.[4] Table 2.1 gives a summary of the recommendations taken from our dietetic guidelines.[12]

Once again local circumstances will dictate which team member will carry out these routine measurements. The most important considerations are that they are carried out

Table 2.1 Recommendations on frequency of monitoring[12]

Measurement	Frequency
Weight	Measured and plotted on growth charts at a minimum of every 6 months Local practice may vary for frequency Those under 2 years will need more regular weights (frequency not agreed)
Standing height/supine length/ alternative height[a]	Measured and plotted on growth charts at a minimum of every 6 months
Triceps skin fold thickness and mid-arm circumference	Measurements taken at a minimum of every 12 months
Dietary assessment and feeding assessment	As required by individual child. Important to review as child enters each age group for recommended nutritional intakes

a. see p. 23.

accurately and regularly reported back to the team or dietitian in overall care of the child's nutrition. Regular multidisciplinary team meetings allow for feedback and highlight any ongoing issues or immediate concerns which can then be dealt with by the most appropriate member/s of the team.

Box 2.4 Frequently asked questions in children with neurological impairment

'I have plotted the child's weight under the 0.4th centile: do they have faltering growth?'
The 0.4th centile on standard reference charts may (depending on the child's age) be above the 50th centile on growth charts specifically for children with cerebral palsy (see Appendix 1). Thus having a recording below the 0.4th centile on the standard charts does not mean the same as it does (significant wasting) in children without cerebral palsy.

It is generally established practice that when a child's weight is under the 0.4th on the Child Growth Foundation growth charts, that this can be acceptable as long as the weights are following the general curve of the centile lines. You should also expect the weight and height to be approximately on the same centile lines.

'We have just started a child on gastrostomy feeding: how do I know I am giving them the right amount of nutrition?'
Many parents are particularly concerned about the child gaining too much weight. We base the initial feeding regime on an estimation of their previous intake with an increase of around 200 kcal per day if they have not been gaining weight. We would then expect to monitor their weight around fortnightly until they are established on their regime; a quick weight gain would indicate a need to reduce the energy intake and no weight gain would indicate the need to increase the energy. For a child with a habitual energy intake below 800 kcal per day we would especially look at their protein intake in their feeding regime.

'What are ideal nutritional indicators and biochemical markers?'
This is an area where paediatric dietitians have been searching for answers for a very long time. It is a question we wished to address when developing our guidelines but because of a lack of evidence in the literature we were unable to make any comment. Our guidelines recommend further research into this area.

'How frequently should children using HETF be reviewed?'
This is a question that is very much open for debate. Our personal opinion, which is not evidence based, is that for children under 1 year of age, monthly review would be ideal; 3-monthly review for 1–5 year olds and 6-monthly reviews for the over 5s, providing they are quite stable. From personal experience we know that this is often not feasible because of limited dietetic resources and local circumstances. Our guidelines (Table 2.1) make some general recommendations for children with neurological impairment who have been referred for faltering growth who may or may not be on HETF.

Conclusion

The nutritional assessment and monitoring of children with neurological impairment are important clinical concerns for health professionals responsible for the medical care of these children. Without a doubt a team of health professionals ideally involving a core group consisting of a consultant paediatrician, specialist paediatric dietitian and specialist paediatric speech and language therapist is the best way to carry this out.

The evidence at this in time is scant and much of what is written in this chapter is based on best current practice and our clinical expertise. The systematic assessment and continuous regular monitoring of these children is important for a number of reasons. The quality of life of the child should always be the over riding goal of any form of medical therapy. Proper nutrition can lead to the child achieving their full growth potential as well as a reducing fatigue, feelings of misery and number of infections. Clinical decisions to introduce special dietary supplements and indeed enteral feeding are based on the recorded weights and heights. Changes to the regimes are often made following subsequent measurements. Indeed a decision by the team to refer a child to child protection agencies can be made on the basis of weight measurements. It is therefore of utmost importance that health professionals should ensure that these measurements are carried out accurately and on a regular basis.

We are sure that in the next few years some of the gaps in the evidence base will be filled. Work is currently being carried out in the UK looking for the most effective alternative method for measuring height in this client group and we would hope that training programmes will be established. With the growth in HETF across the UK work is also being carried out looking at the most appropriate biochemical and haematological indices required for monitoring these children.

References

1. Vedantham S, Taylor FC, Yousefzadeh DK, Udekwu P, Thistlethwaite JR, Whitington PF. Abdominal pain in a young girl due to congenital stenosis of the common bile duct with mucus plug formation. *J Pediatr Gastroenterol Nutr* 1992; **15**: 440–3.
2. Stevenson RD. Measurement of growth in children with developmental disabilities. *Dev Med Child Neurol* 1996; **38**: 855–60.
3. Spender QW, Cronk CE, Charney EB, Stallings VA. Assessment of linear growth of children with cerebral palsy: use of alternative measures to height or length [published erratum appears in Dev Med Child Neurol 1990; 32: 1032]. *Dev Med Child Neurol* 1989; **31**: 206–14
4. Stallings VA, Cronk CE, Zemel BS, Charney EB. Body composition in children with spastic quadriplegic cerebral palsy. *J Pediatr* 1995; **126**: 833–9.
5. Stallings VA, Charney EB, Davies JC, Cronk CE. Nutritional status and growth of children with diplegic or hemiplegic cerebral palsy. *Dev Med Child Neurol* 1993; **35**: 997–1006.
6. Stevenson RD. Use of segmental measures to estimate stature in children with cerebral palsy. *Arch Pediatr Adolesc Med* 1995; **149**: 658–62.
7. Stewart L, McKaig N, Dunlop C, Daly H, Almond S. Assessment and monitoring of children with neurodisability on home enteral tube feeding. *Clinical Nutrition Update* 2005; **10**: 6–8.
8. Krick J, Murphy-Miller P, Zeger S, Wright E. Pattern of growth in children with cerebral palsy. *J Am Diet Assoc* 1996; **96**: 680–5.
9. Samson-Fang LJ, Stevenson RD. Identification of malnutrition in children with cerebral palsy: poor performance of weight-for-height centiles. *Dev Med Child Neurol* 2000; **42**: 162–8.
10. Frisancho AR. New norms of upper limb fat and muscle areas for assessment of nutritional status. *Am J Clin Nutr* 1981; **34**: 2540–5.
11. Sullivan PB, Juszczak E, Lambert BR, Rose M, Ford-Adams ME, Johnson A. Impact of feeding problems on nutritional intake and growth: Oxford Feeding Study II. *Dev Med Child Neurol* 2002; **44**: 461–7.
12. Stewart L, McKaig N, Dunlop C, Almond S. *Guidelines on dietetic assessment and monitoring of children with special needs with faltering growth.* British Dietetic Association, 2006. Available from: http://www.bda.co.uk
13. Stallings, VA, Zemel BS, Davies JC, Cronk CE, Charney EB. Energy expenditure of children and adolescents with severe disabilities: a cerebral palsy model. *Am J Clin Nutr* 1996; **64**: 627–34.
14. Troughton KE, Hill AE. Relation between objectively measured feeding competence and nutrition in children with cerebral palsy. *Dev Med Child Neurol* 2001; **43**: 187–90.
15. Fung EB, Samson-Fang L, Stallings VA et al. Feeding dysfunction is associated with poor growth and health status in children with cerebral palsy. *J Am Diet Assoc* 2002; **102**: 3–73.
16. Todorovic VMA. *A Pocket Guide to Clinical Nutrition*, 2nd edn. London: Parenteral and Enteral Nutrition Group of the British Dietetic Association; 2000.
17. NHS Lothain. *Lothian Enteral Tube Feeding Best Practice Statement for Adults and Children.* Edinburgh: NHS Lothian, 2007.

18. Thomas AG, Akobeng AK. Technical aspects of feeding the disabled child. *Curr Opin Clin Nutr Metab Care* 2000; 3: 221–5.

19. Dietary reference values for food energy and nutrients for the United Kingdom. *Report of the Panel on Dietary Reference Values of the Committee on Medical Aspects of Food Policy*, 41th edn. London: HMSO, 1991.

20. Dietetic Department, Great Ormond Street Hospital. *Nutritional Requirements for Children in Health and Disease*, 3rd edn. London: Great Ormond Street Hospital for Children NHS Trust, 2000.

21. A Committee of the British Association for Parental and Enteral Nutrition. *Trends in Artificial Nutrition Support in the UK between 1996 and 2002. A Report by the British Artificial Nutrition Survey*. Redditch: BANS, 2003.

Acknowledgements

We would like to thank Hilary Daly, Carolyn Dunlop and Sarah Almond for their work on the dietetic guidelines on the assessment and monitoring of children with special needs who are failing to thrive, which underpinned much of this chapter.

We thank Sarah Almond kindly allowing us to reproduce photographs showing the alternative height measurements.

Chapter 3

Oral Motor Impairment and Swallowing Dysfunction: Assessment and management

Sue Strudwick

Introduction

Children with neurological impairment commonly have oral motor difficulties and, as a result, many have feeding difficulties; the incidence varies from 30 to 81%.[1,2]

It is well documented that, of these children, those with oropharyngeal impairments are also likely to aspirate, which is a major cause of morbidity and mortality. The prevalence of aspiration in children with severe neurodisability is as high as 68–70%.[3,4] Feeding is a complex task which requires motor and sensory pathway integration and significant neuromuscular coordination.[5] It is therefore essential to carry out a thorough assessment of a child's eating and drinking skills, in order to determine the risks of aspiration and select management strategies to maximize safety, nutrition and hydration for these children.

Children with neurological impairment present with differing problems associated with eating and drinking. There are those who manage to eat and drink safely, possibly with significant support from a parent/carer, but for whom the effort and poor oropharyngeal skills reduce the efficiency of intake. This has adverse effects on nutrition and hydration status. Even those children with relatively mild eating and drinking dysfunction may be at risk of poor nutritional status.[1]

Some children have such significant oropharyngeal difficulties and swallowing problems that their swallow is unsafe and they are unable to protect their airway leading to chest infections and increased morbidity and mortality.[6,7] These two scenarios are not the only permutation of eating and drinking difficulties, but have been chosen to demonstrate the importance of a comprehensive assessment in order to plan the most effective management and to eliminate risk wherever possible.

Both these scenarios can be extremely distressing for the child, his family and his carers. It is not just the safety issue that should be addressed in the assessment of a child's eating and drinking skills but also the wider impact of the effect on the child and family.

It is not sufficient to undertake an assessment that only considers aspiration and safety. The effect of the eating and drinking difficulties on nutrition, hydration and quality of life should also be given great importance.

The assessment of eating and drinking

The speech and language therapist (SLT) should undertake an eating and drinking assessment in order to:[8,9]

- assess and maximize swallow safety;
- identify potential risk;
- maximize the child's eating and drinking potential;
- reduce anxiety and distress around eating and drinking;
- help the child and carers to make decisions around feeding options when oral intake alone may not be possible;
- plan management strategies;
- support the child and carers and increase their knowledge of their child's eating and drinking difficulties.

The assessment

Gross motor skills

The greater the degree of motor impairment, the more likely there will be eating and drinking problems and nutritional issues.[10] Postural management is known to reduce risk and improve feeding;[11] therefore, it is vital to look at gross motor skills. The child's ability to control movement, their tone – hypertonia or hypotonia and/or a mixture, their stability, symmetry, degree of independence, and most importantly, head control, must all be carefully assessed.

The SLT should have experience of working with children with a neurodevelopmental disability; nevertheless it is essential that the multidisciplinary team be involved here as is emphasized in other chapters.

The physiotherapist and occupational therapist should be consulted and a joint assessment should take place with a specific emphasis on skills for eating and drinking. Their expertise will inform advice on postural control and seating.

The SLT will be able to identify which aspects of the child's positioning are likely to impede safe and effective eating and drinking. The presence of any reflexes (either abnormal or persistent primitive) should also be noted. The asymmetrical tonic neck reflex when the child's head turns away from his flexed arm (such as is required for self-feeding) is an example of a reflex that can have a significant impact on eating and drinking. The persistence of these reflexes can preclude the development of useful, voluntary movements.

Head control is the most important postural influence on eating and drinking. The position of the head in relation to the rest of the body will impinge on the safety of swallow.[12] For instance, if the head is not in the midline it will be more difficult for the child to swallow with control and to maintain the airway safely. If the head is tilted back the airway remains open and unprotected; if the head is too far forward the airway may become occluded, thereby making the swallow more difficult. Thus, children with a neurological impairment often have an impaired swallow which will be exacerbated by a poor head position. Reduced laryngeal elevation has been cited as a significant cause of aspiration, often caused by neck extension.[13] Careful head and neck positioning is essential to promote safe feeding in children with neurological impairment.

Effort involved in maintaining head control also plays a part. If it is hard for the child to hold their head up, how can the finer tuned internal muscles required for eating and swallowing work? The effort may well result in fatigue, which will also impair control.

Strauss et al (1997) noted that those children who could not lift their heads and were tube fed were most at risk of early death in early childhood.[12] This study concurs with that of Morton et al (2002).[13]

Seating/positioning

The assessment should also include how the child is seated for eating and drinking. This may differ from seating for other activities. The child may also have the right equipment but not be using it appropriately.

Carers/parents may not be aware of the difference that a slight change in the angle of the child's head or the angle of his or her body posture makes on the child's function for eating and drinking. The aim is to achieve stability and symmetry (Figure 3.1). The child should ideally be positioned with their hips and knees at right angles to their body. This will involve an assessment of joint mobility particularly of the hips, knees and ankles, shoulders and spine. The child needs proximal stability to achieve distal mobility. Their head should be in the midline, with a slight chin tuck, and with no extension in the neck. Their shoulders should be slightly flexed. Reflexes that increase extension of the trunk and head may increase the risk of aspiration.

The occupational therapist will advise on different options for seating or standing for eating and drinking. Access to suitable seating varies according to funding and locality.

The child may have a very carefully designed chair for school, but this may not travel home and therefore the seating at home may be less than ideal. Similarly, the child may

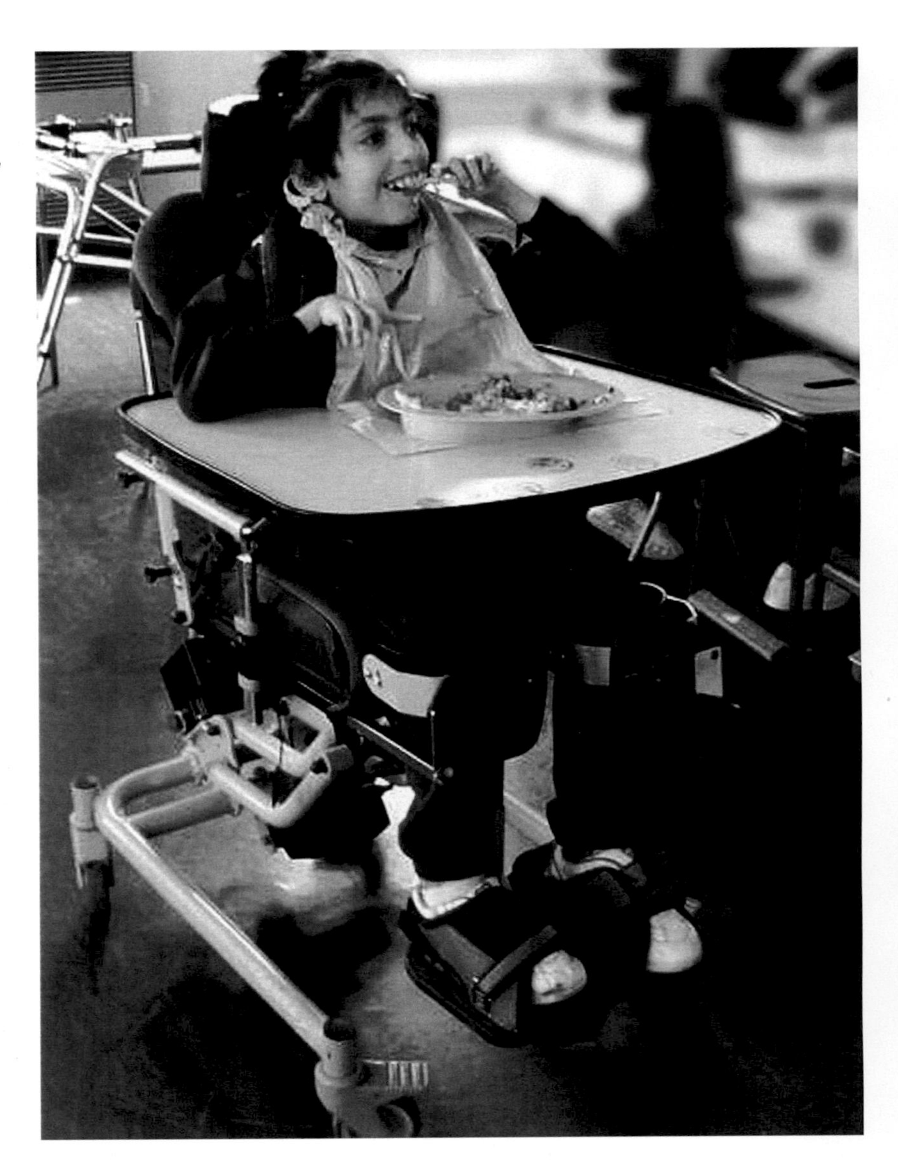

Figure 3.1 A child in a supportive seating system, self-feeding.

have respite care, but that centre may not have appropriate seating. This will increase the risk of eating and drinking difficulties and the potential risk of aspiration.This also underlines the need to have a full picture of the child's ability to eat and drink in all settings and to be aware of compromises that may be being made when there is no suitable chair. As children grow and their needs change, regular reviews of the suitability of the seating are essential to maintain the best position for eating and drinking.

The position of the person feeding the dependent children can also positively or negatively impact on positioning, oral motor skills and swallow safety (see Management strategies below). Asking the advice of an occupational therapist is essential.

Oral motor skills

Oral motor function is a highly complex, multiskilled task and careful assessment by an experienced clinician remains the only effective way of measuring oral motor function and its impact on eating and drinking.

Prior to the assessment, the SLT will gather information from appropriate sources in order to decide which assessments to carry out; a useful resource is the Clinical Guidelines produced by the Royal College of Speech and Language Therapists (RCSLT).[8] This will enable a preliminary assessment of risk to be undertaken.

The SLT should undertake a thorough assessment of a child's oral motor skills as part of the feeding assessment. In typically developing children, there is a dynamic interplay between the child's oral motor skill development and the opportunity to practise it in feeding. The child with very poor oral motor skills and unsafe swallow will have missed out on this interplay.

The child's oral motor skills should be evaluated at rest and with the child feeding, ideally in different settings, e.g. school and home, and should include different textures of food and drink.

The Schedule for Oral Motor Assessment can be useful as it is a standardized tool for assessing oral motor skills.[14] However, in the case of children with a marked neurological impairment, it may not always be appropriate and an adapted assessment will be necessary. Various other tools exist[15–17] but the lack of a simple, validated screening tool specifically for this population is recognized.[1] The following should all be assessed.

Jaw

The SLT should observe the physical appearance of the jaw. Many children with cerebral palsy have over bites (the maxillary teeth protruding over the mandibular incisors)[18] that will adversely affect their biting and chewing in addition to their poor oral motor skills.

Tonic biting (biting down hard) may occur at the touch of the spoon. This is unpleasant for the child and the feeder. The child may become very distressed by attempts to get him to release the spoon and this is only likely to increase the bite. This interferes with feeding at all levels.

Jaw stability is important for the child to grade the opening and closing of the mouth appropriately. Poor jaw stability will lead to poor grading, which in turn causes ineffective ability to manipulate the food in the oral cavity, poor bolus formation and swallowing, particularly in drinking.

Jaw thrusting can be observed as a symptom of poor jaw grading. It is usually seen in children with increased tone.

Jaw retraction may also be associated with increased tone. Both abnormal jaw movements will affect the child's ability to take food off a spoon or drink from a cup, beaker or bottle. It will also affect their ability to hold the food or fluid in the mouth, to manipulate it, to form a bolus and to swallow effectively and safely. Management of the jaw movements forms a core part of the SLT's eating and drinking plan.

Lips
First, observation of the child's lip position at rest is necessary.

- Are the lips together at rest or apart?
- What is the tone of the child's lips?
- Is there sign of low tone, hypotonia with flaccid looking lips?
- Is there evidence of increased tone, hypertonia, with pursing or retraction?
- Is there evidence of mixed tone and athetoid movements with the lips constantly moving at rest?

The same observations then need to be undertaken during eating and drinking.

The functional movement should be observed, evaluating the ability of the child to take the food off the spoon or fork, particularly with the upper lip.

- Can the child bring their lips together in order to keep the food in the oral cavity?
- Are the lips together, producing negative intra-oral pressure for an effective swallow?

It is important to note the timing of this, as the child may have the ability to achieve lip closure, but may not have the fine motor skill to carry out the movement quickly.

Effective eating and drinking is the result of sequential movements, carried out quickly. Poor control will lead to food or fluid loss with its consequences of poor nutrition and dehydration.[1]

There may be asymmetrical lip movements that will also have an effect on the ability of the child to take the food off the spoon or liquid out of the cup. Asymmetrical movements may lead to increased effort to maintain function, with the implication of fatigue reducing both safety and successful eating and drinking. Lack of consistent lip closure may also lead to drooling, which will be discussed later in the chapter.

Cheeks
The movements of the cheeks during the oral phase of eating and drinking will show whether they are playing their part in containing and moving the bolus inside the mouth. The cheeks support lip and tongue movement. Lack of tone in the cheeks can lead to food collecting in the lateral sulci, thereby reducing the ability of the child to form a cohesive bolus for swallowing.

Tongue
Typically developing children will demonstrate tongue movements in the order of horizontal, vertical and lateral, the latter appearing at around 9 months.[19,20] This development will allow children to cope with lumps more effectively, by chewing –moving the food around between the biting surfaces on either side of the mouth, crossing the midline and then retrieving the food back into the midline to form a bolus. Many children with abnormal neurological development will not have developed lateral tongue movements. They will not be able to chew effectively. It is essential that the SLT assesses these tongue movements in particular, as they will have significant consequences for the textures that the child can safely cope with.

The tongue's appearance at rest should initially be noted. The tongue may be hypotonic and lie flat on the bottom of the mouth. In contrast, it may be hypertonic with a bunched appearance. It is important to note asymmetry and fasciculation as indicators of the type of damage to the cranial nerves.

Tongue thrusting is very common in children with cerebral palsy. This clearly leads to food loss as well as compromised ability to form and manipulate a bolus. Spoon and cup placement is also difficult with a strong tongue thrust. Tongue retraction may be observed.

Limited tongue movement results in poor control of the food, slow or ineffective bolus formation, poor oral transit backwards in preparation for the swallow and an inability to manipulate the food for chewing. The back of the tongue needs to rise in order to effect a swallow. This will be discussed in the pharyngeal/swallowing assessment.

Incoordination of the components of oral motor function is perhaps the most significant aspect to consider when assessing these skills for eating and drinking.

Effective and safe feeding patterns consist of rhythmical, sequential, carefully timed movements.[21] The timing, speed, intensity and interplay of movement are crucial in evaluating the total pattern in relation to eating and drinking.

The sum of the parts is not always the same as the whole and what is assessed and recorded about the child's oral motor skills does not necessarily match what one sees at functional mealtimes. There are many things that influence the mealtime process which will be discussed later. All need to be taken into account.

Swallowing
There are four phases of swallowing: oral preparatory, oral , pharyngeal and oesophageal.[22] Swallowing involves the preparation of the food, the formation of the bolus, oral transit and then propulsion of the bolus through the pharyngeal area with the airway protected. When the fine-tuning of this process fails, aspiration is likely to follow.

It is necessary to distinguish between aspiration and penetration. Penetration occurs when foreign material passes into the laryngeal vestibule but not below the true vocal cords. Aspiration occurs when foreign material passes into the laryngeal vestibule and passes below the vocal cords into the trachea and lungs.[22] Aspiration can be of food, liquid or secretions (primary aspiration) or refluxate from the stomach (secondary aspiration). The incidence of aspiration in the child with neurological impairment is very high and has been shown to occur in 68–70% of children with severe disability.[3,4]

Aspiration can be:

- chronic (long term) or acute (sudden onset);
- silent – no coughing or choking;
- associated with respiratory problems;
- associated with fatigue at the end of feeds;
- secondary to gastro-oesophageal reflux;
- mild, moderate, severe or profound.[23]

Causes and contributory factors include:

- poor tongue and oral movements, leading to poor collection of food in the mouth;
- inappropriate textures being offered;
- inappropriate pacing and amount offered;
- poor pharyngeal movements;
- inadequate clearing of the pharyngeal area;
- reduced laryngeal elevation and closure;
- delayed/absent swallow reflex;
- poor coordination of swallowing and breathing;
- state levels: arousal/stress;
- poor control of reflux;
- respiratory disease, including colds and coughs.

The result of aspiration is difficult to predict. One study has shown that the amount and frequency of aspiration does not necessarily directly relate to lung damage.[24] Nevertheless, there are numerous studies showing that children who aspirate are at risk of chest infections, poor nutrition and concomitant morbidity and mortality.[6,10,25,26]

Fatigue can play a major part in aspiration, particularly in children with neurological impairment. A child may be safe at the beginning of the meal but the effort of managing the food and/or drink can lead to fatigue, less coordination and greater risk of aspiration. This must be accounted for in the course of a meal and the day as a whole.

There are recent developments in assessing the airways of children with cerebral palsy. Upper airway obstruction may also be a component of aspiration risk.

Assessment of aspiration

Clinical evaluation is extremely important in assessing the possibility of aspiration but it is not possible to be absolutely accurate from clinical evidence alone. DeMatteo et al compared the clinical evaluation with that of videofluoroscopy to detect aspiration.[27] Interestingly, there was much greater accuracy in clinically detecting aspiration of fluids where 92% sensitivity was found. In detecting aspiration with solids, accuracy dropped to 33%. The majority of children were aged less than 12 months. Cough was the most significant predictor of fluid aspiration and penetration. There was a higher incidence of aspiration on fluids – 40% prevalence for fluids and 18% for solids in the sample of 75 children. Aspiration with liquids and solids may not be accurately predicted from clinical evaluation alone. This endorses the need for videofluoroscopy (VFSS) as an evaluative tool.[28,29]

Observations of clinical signs of aspiration are essential to note and monitor in order to evaluate risk and plan management. Clinical signs are:[19,30]

- history of chest infections;
- inability to handle own secretions;
- coughing or choking during/after feeds;
- very poor oral motor coordination;
- delayed swallow reflex;
- multiple swallows to clear single bolus;
- limited endurance/increasing fatigue;
- noisy/wet upper airway sounds during or after feeding;
- wet voice quality during/after feeding;
- apnoea or increased congestion during feeds;
- change in breathing rhythm;
- blinking, eyes watering;
- throat clearing, grimacing, head tilting.

Other warning signs include gagging, long periods chewing food, stringy mucous, refusal of food/drink, poor oral hygiene, taking a long time to eat a meal, low body weight/weight loss, dehydration.[31]

These signs and the total picture of the child's eating and drinking can be assessed and a risk form completed to inform management of the risk and the need to refer on for VFS. The various aspects of the whole pattern of eating and drinking can be evaluated in terms of risk and actions taken to reduce that risk. The form below (Figure 3.1) is currently being trialled for accuracy and clinical viability as part of a comprehensive risk assessment tool.

As described earlier, aspiration can occur as 'silent aspiration' with no overt or protective signs at all.[3,4,28,32] In Arvedson's study, of those who aspirated, almost all – 94% – had silent aspiration.[28] It is this aspect of aspiration that warrants most attention.

ASSESSMENT OF EATING AND DRINKING SKILLS

Name of Child:............ Date:............ Place:............
Dob:............ Time:............ Person Assisting:............
What the meal is:............ Length of Meal:............ Dependent/independent:............
Is this typical:............ Initial Assessment ☐ Reassessment ☐

Factors to consider:	Eating Assessment:	Drinking Assessment:	Risk Factor
1. Child Positioning/Seating			☐ ☐
2. Position of Feeder			☐ ☐
3. Utensils used eg. bottle, cup , etc			☐ ☐
4. Texture of food/drink			☐ ☐
5. Size of mouthful/sips			☐ ☐
6. Pacing			☐ ☐
7. Oral skills (lips, tongue, cheeks, palate, jaw, teeth)			☐ ☐
8. Swallow			☐ ☐
9. Specific difficulties, eg. Gagging, reflux, respiratory status, signs of aspiration			☐ ☐
10. Degree of assistance eg. Oral control, hand over hand			☐ ☐
11. Communcation and Behaviour			☐ ☐

RISK ASSESSMENT OF EATING AND DRINKING

12. Signs of Aspiration:

- ☐ History of chest infections
- ☐ Inability to handle own secretions
- ☐ Coughing or choking during/after feeds
- ☐ Very poor oro-motor co-ordination
- ☐ Delayed swallow
- ☐ Multiple swallows to clear single bollus
- ☐ Limited endurance
- ☐ Noisy/wet upper airways sounds during/after feeding
- ☐ Wet voice quality during/after feeding
- ☐ Apnoea or increased congestion during feeds
- ☐ Change in breathing rhythm – faster or slower or both
- ☐ Change in colour, note particular lips
- ☐ Blinking/eye widening/eye watering
- ☐ Throat clearing
- ☐ Grimaching
- ☐ Head tilting
- ☐ Arching during feed

Risk Factors:	Severe	Mod	Mild	Action to reduce risk	Outcome Sev	Med	Mild
	☐	☐	☐		☐	☐	☐

Information from history:

Information from parents/carer:

Recommendations/objectives:

Feeding category =
Prioritisation:

Signed: ____________________
Speech and Language Therapist

Figure 3.2 Assessment of eating and drinking skills.

It is not sufficient for the clinician to look for overt signs of aspiration or to look for other signs such as chest infections, as these may not be present despite the child aspirating silently.

Where there are concerns about the child's feeding, assessment should be undertaken carefully, clinical risk evaluated and suitable treatment options planned, together with honest discussion with parents about the risks and benefits of oral feeding.

Cervical auscultation is being used more frequently as a tool in assessing pharyngeal swallows. The interpretation of the sounds relies on the experience of the clinician. A stethoscope is placed on the side of the larynx and breath sounds are evaluated before, during and after the swallow.

The RCSLT Clinical Guidelines (2005) state that cervical auscultation should not be the sole tool of assessment of aspiration.[8] However, there are further studies[33] indicating the development of a more objective interpretation of acoustic data and use of acoustic information to aid detection of aspiration in a non-invasive way.

Cervical auscultation is a readily accessible tool, particularly for those clinicians working in the community, including schools and children's homes. It is non-invasive. It should be used in conjunction with good clinical assessment and should inform clinicians of further investigations that may be necessary.

Videofluoroscopy
Videofluoroscopy (VFS) is an invaluable tool as part of the clinical assessment of the child with neurological impairment. VFS can show the visual representation of the physiology and function of the anatomical structures and how they interact during eating and/or drinking.

Arvedson et al describes the use of VFS and the interpretation of the timing of the swallow in excellent detail.[30] From the clinician's point of view, the findings of the VFS need careful evaluation in order to inform practice. It is very important to show where and when aspiration or penetration occurs as this will inform our intervention and whether it will be possible for the child to be able to eat and/or drink safely. For instance, the lack of clearance from the pharyngeal area (pharyngeal delay) and reduced laryngeal elevation are important determinants of aspiration.[13] Pharyngeal delay increases the time the food lingers in the pharynx, thereby increasing the risk of aspiration before the swallow. Reduced laryngeal elevation prevents pharyngeal clearance, thus allowing for aspiration after the swallow. This study[13] highlighted the influence the respiratory pattern, particularly inspiration, has on the risk of aspiration. As has been highlighted before, the position of the head and neck is crucial in reducing this risk.

VFS is more than just a tool for identifying aspiration. The VFS can assist decisions regarding optimal feeding position, rate of feeding and suitable textures[34] and a suitable feeding plan can be agreed.

Access to VFS is restricted in the UK because many local centres and hospitals do not have a VFS suite. In practical terms, this tends to lead to only small numbers of children being referred – often those who clearly have clinical signs of oral motor impairment and swallowing dysfunction, whereas there are many more children who would be managed better if the SLT had access to VFS.

Interpretation of the findings of VFS should be used in conjunction with the clinical picture in order to prioritize and plan effective intervention. VFS can be a very informative investigation for parents and carers. Until they see the results of the VFS, many parents find it hard to believe that their child is aspirating or at risk of aspiration. Many of these children may not have had significant chest infections. The parents/carers may have limited or no knowledge of the anatomy and physiology of eating and drinking and 'it goes down the wrong way' may be understood as a common feature of everyday life without the perspective of the potential damage and life-threatening consequences.

It may be that feeding orally may not be a safe option. Careful discussion with the team, undertaken within the framework of the parental perspective, is essential.

The weighing up of the risks versus benefits of oral feeding is nearly always emotive and ethically challenging. Protection of the child and acting in the child's best interests is the SLT's paramount duty. But this should be carried out with sympathy and respect for the parents who, in most cases, feed their child everyday. In practice, preparation for the VFS is all important. Using it as a way of making the parents take note of the SLT's advice rarely brings about the expected outcome. A careful discussion about why the procedure is being carried out and what might be found is important, as are the possible consequences for management.

Unless the discussion takes place as a team, the parents can find themselves in the invidious position of hearing conflicting advice from the professionals most closely involved with their child. This situation is not a rare occurrence and parents cite this as being most distressing in trying to decide for themselves what is the best course of action for their child.[35]

Other important issues

As well as position, oral motor skills, and the pharyngeal stage of swallowing, there are other considerations that should be taken into account when the SLT is assessing the child's eating and drinking.

Communication

The child and carer's interaction and communication is vital to the success of the eating and drinking process. The child's preferred method of communication should always be employed and responded to, at the mealtime. The interaction between the feeder and the child is all-important in trying to achieve a safe, enjoyable experience for the child. The child may need cueing in for each mouthful;

the feeder will need to regulate the pacing of the mouthfuls; the child may need augmentative communication strategies such as symbols, photographs etc. in order to make choices and indicate readiness or otherwise. Consistency between feeders, particularly at home and in school can be difficult, but should form part of the feeding plan.

Environment

The SLT should take into account the effect of the environment in terms of visual and noise distraction. External influences can disorganize oral movements.

Alertness can affect the eating and drinking process positively or negatively. The child who is distracted by sights and sounds may attempt to turn their head to see what is happening or perhaps going into extension at the sudden noises heard. Either scenario lessens the control the child has over their head and neck position and therefore reduces safety. Extensor spasms or movements have been strongly linked with aspiration.[13] The balance of social involvement with safe eating and drinking needs to be carefully measured. Lack of alertness may lead to the child being unable to take a proactive role in eating and drinking. He will have less control over the fine motor skills involved with eating and drinking and will be less communicative, thereby leaving him more vulnerable to inappropriate feeding.

Medication

Medication, for example anti-epileptic or antidrooling medication, may affect alertness, appetite, and dryness of mouth, amongst other symptoms. It is important therefore to note the medication the child is on and the effect it is likely to have on eating and drinking.

Vision

If the child is visually impaired, they will be less able to anticipate the food coming and will not see what they are going to eat or drink. Time, cueing, consistency and preparation will all need to be considered for the visually impaired child.[19]

Gastro-oesophageal reflux

Often under diagnosed, GOR is very common in children with neurological impairment.[2,36]

Its impact in this population cannot be overemphasized. Food refusal, pain, nausea, lack of appetite/interest in food, aspiration of gastric contents, all can be attributed to reflux but are commonly attributed to 'behaviour', the oropharyngeal difficulties, or the abnormal tone of the neurological impairment itself e.g. extensor spasms versus arching in pain.

Further investigation of the possible presence of reflux is essential in obtaining a total view of the eating and drinking process for any individual child (See Chapter 6).

Constipation
Constipation also significantly affects eating and drinking (see Chapter 6).

Cognitive level of the child
The child's awareness of the mealtime experience, his/her ability to understand the language used and to interpret various signals – communicative, visual and auditory – will all play a part in the eating and drinking experience. Parental expectations and prognosis of the condition will also influence strategies, plans and expected outcomes of intervention.

Behaviour
Some children with neurological impairment show aversive feeding behaviours. The reasons for negative associations with mealtimes should be fully assessed wherever possible. Reflux, pain, fear, sensory issues, past unpleasant mealtimes and past negative experiences must be evaluated so that appropriate strategies are put in place. The clinician needs to consider behavioural issues, because refusal of food means that any feeding plan cannot be implemented. Looking at possible causes is the first step. Consistencies of approach and good evidence-based strategies are needed. Feeding is an interactive and reciprocal activity. This interaction can easily break down when the child has difficulties in eating and drinking. The child's cues are often missed or ignored because of the carer's anxiety about safety or getting the child to take 'enough' food.

The child with neurological impairment is especially vulnerable to maladaption to changes and transitions to different textures. Their lack of autonomy compounds this.[37] These children can be very cautious or even fearful of new situations in feeding. The SLT should take a very good history, including any reference to gastro-oesophageal reflux. This can have a profound influence on feeding, leading to food refusal, poor interaction during feeding, and gagging.[38] These behaviours are often misinterpreted as the child being difficult. Equally, pain from constipation, fear of aspiration, discomfort when eating and drinking and effortful eating will all contribute to an unpleasant experience for the child. This is likely only to worsen if the causes are not recognized and dealt with appropriately. Interventions such as nasogastric feeds, and suctioning, which may have been used in the past, can impair the development of normal feeding patterns.[39] Cognisance of the causes of behaviours should inform the SLT about trying to reduce the negative influences on eating and drinking.

The SLT can also help to reduce these behaviours by implementing good feeding practice. Force feeding should always be avoided, and pausing, following the child's cues, increasing interaction and encouragement are all significant behavioural strategies that should be employed.[40] Wherever possible, children should be given autonomy in eating and drinking, although this can be difficult to achieve in the totally dependent child. Utilizing communication aids, responding to non-verbal cues, and giving choices are all important approaches that can increase autonomy and control for children. Behavioural interventions apply equally to children with a neurological impairment as to those without; yet, in practice, this aspect of eating and drinking is often neglected or not given sufficient emphasis.

If good feeding practices do not resolve the situation, then referral to a clinical psychologist should be considered. In all cases, consistency of approach across all settings is crucial. Gastrostomy feeding may not alleviate carers' attitudes to or perceptions of eating and drinking. The psychosocial aspects of eating and drinking are complex and should be given due importance in managing any behavioural issues.[41]

Oral hygiene and sensitivity

Children with poor oral motor skills often have abnormal oral sensory reactions and these can affect the feeding process, especially if there is a strong gag response, or particular hypersensitivity to temperature, taste and texture. Oral hygiene and in particular, mouth ulcers, oral thrush, dental caries and periodontal disease should be investigated, in order to evaluate whether oral discomfort is contributing to the dysfunctional eating and drinking. Oral hygiene tends to be compromised in children who mouth breath and drool.

Management strategies

Respect for parents' perspectives and real collaboration between parents and professionals is key to successful implementation of any plan. The SLT's initial aim, following a thorough assessment, is to reduce the risk of aspiration, dehydration and poor nutrition. Therefore, with close involvement of the parents as an integral part of the multidisciplinary team, we should be endeavouring to maximize nutrition, hydration and safety and enhance the mealtime experience for the child and family.

An eating and drinking plan should be formulated for each child and disseminated to all who are involved with the child.[8]

Position of the child and carer

Together with the physiotherapist and occupational therapist, the child's seating must be adapted in order to maximize stability, to normalize tone if possible, to minimize abnormal reflexes and to give good head control. The child's head position should ideally be with slightly flexed shoulders, a slight chin tuck and an elongated back of the neck. Caution is necessary to ensure the airway is not occluded for breathing.

The person feeding the child can put their hand on the child's head in order to offer support but this should be demonstrated first as it can lead to pushing the head down and back, therefore reducing laryngeal elevation and increasing the risk of aspiration.[42] Shoulder stability is essential in maintaining a good head position and maximizing oropharyngeal skills. A tray may be useful to support and stabilize the arms and shoulders. Some children eat well in a standing frame.

The person feeding the child needs to be in a position where they can see the child's face, to observe signs of aspiration and respond appropriately to the child's verbal or non-verbal communication. They also need to be at the right height so that the child does not need to turn their head, thus changing head position, or raise their eyes, as this will tilt their head back, thus increasing the potential for aspiration. Care of the feeder's back should also be taken into consideration both in terms of their back health and in terms of offering the best feeding technique they can for the child.

Texture/diet modification

The texture of the food and drink should reflect the child's ability to cope with that texture. A comprehensive assessment of the child's oropharyngeal skills will inform this part of the feeding plan. If a child has no lateral tongue movements and is unable to manipulate the food between the biting surfaces and back to the centre as a bolus for swallowing, they should not be offered food that requires chewing. It may be that the child can only deal safely with a smooth puréed consistency. The thickness or viscosity of the purée should also be defined. Mixed textures are the most difficult to manipulate orally so should be avoided in the child with oral motor difficulties. Foods can be mashed or puréed but should be selected according to the ability of each child to cope with the specific texture. SLTs have devised a Guide to Textures to help with this selection.[43]

Oral transit time must also be considered. Anterior loss of food/drink clearly leads to nutritional risks, but preventing this by thickening may mean that oral transit is reduced and the child is unable to move the bolus back efficiently for swallowing. This can lead to gagging and/or aspiration. A balance needs to be achieved, with safety being the most important factor. The optimal texture needs to be trialled and agreed. Some children will be able to chew, but again, optimal texture should be agreed. Parents are often very keen to move their children on to more challenging textures. More demanding textures take more time to chew and may lead to greater fatigue and less safe swallowing. The advantages of offering more challenging textures should always be examined against the risk of compromising swallow safety.

In many, but not all children with neurological impairment, thin liquids are the most likely to cause aspiration. Thickening fluid to syrup or custard consistency will give more sensory feedback within the mouth and give the child additional time to control the swallow as well as better respiratory control.[44,45]

Technique

How the food/drink is delivered, including the pacing and amount on the spoon or tipped from the cup can improve the eating and drinking process and thereby both safety and intake.[19,46] Pinnington's study using a Robotic Aid to Eating showed that consistent presentation positively improved the feeding process but was difficult to sustain and artificial.[47] In practice, signs of increased distress, less control and poorer oropharyngeal skills can be noted when observing inconsistent and inappropriate feeding techniques.

Rushing the process by giving another spoonful when the child has not cleared the previous one can lead to a lack of control, overfilling of the mouth, resulting in distress to the child and possible aspiration.

Good observations and communication between the child and the person feeding the child are vital in determining the timing and regulating the respiratory rate. The person feeding the child carries the responsibility for ensuring that the child is fed at a safe pace, with sufficient but small enough amounts to be safely dealt with and time to prepare for the next mouthful or sip of drink.[13,45]

The length of the meal may well be affected both by allowing sufficient timing for each mouthful but also by the presentation of more challenging textures. Providing greater calorie density can keep the meal, and therefore fatigue, within reasonable limits. Working together with the dietitian is paramount to good management.

Oral control
Control of the mouth, jaw, cheeks and lips can be significantly improved through hands-on oral control by a trained therapist/carer. It can inhibit reflexes, aid lip closure, jaw stability and facilitate graded movement as well as reducing abnormal movements. Often, children with neurological impairment have poor jaw grading and appropriate support for the jaw can facilitate good closure on the drinking vessel, better bolus control and safer swallowing. It has been well established that jaw stability is important for effective drinking. It must be considered however, whether giving oral control exacerbates the lack of swallowing control, particularly with fluids. The child may not be able to cope with an increased amount of fluid in the mouth and aspiration can increase as the fluid pours over the back of the tongue before the swallow is triggered. A balance of good oral control versus swallow control should be reached, but safety of the child is paramount.

All oral control techniques should be introduced away from the mealtime, to allow for desensitization and acceptance of the carer's hands on the child's face.

Utensils
The choice of suitable utensils is essential in assisting the person feeding the child achieve efficient and effective safe feeding. The shape, size and material of the spoon need to be planned, having evaluated oral motor skills. Most children with eating and drinking difficulties are better with plastic spoons, but using age appropriate cutlery may be feasible. Drinking vessels, if properly chosen and used, will enable the child to control the fluid better. Cut-away cups made of flexible plastic with space for the nose, enable the feeder to see exactly how the fluid is being delivered and prevents the child from tipping his head back to get the drink.

Choices need to be made on an individual basis, always balancing efficiency and safety. Choosing cups or bottles should involve a careful evaluation of the effect using that vessel will have on the amount of fluid taken.

Many children with neurological impairment suffer from constipation and dehydration, exacerbated by poor intake of fluid. The child's oral motor skills and swallow will impact significantly on his ability to take liquids.

Oral sensorimotor therapy

Oral sensorimotor therapy is widely used by SLTs in clinical practice. Good, consistent oral sensorimotor treatment such as alerting therapy for hypotonia – fast tapping, brushing and stroking, or calming therapy for hypertonia – facial massage, vibration and deep pressure, can help with the day to day management of eating and drinking. Oral stimulation as a preparation for eating and drinking should preferably be followed by oral motor practice with appropriate food and drink, if safe. Developing chewing skills, if safe, can be done with pouches of food and non-food items e.g. specifically designed oral motor tool such as Chewy Tubes. Small changes can make big differences in the child's management of eating and drinking. For instance, helping the child develop some upper lip control can help with removal of the food off the spoon and can help create a good lip seal on the drinking vessel, as well as creating a more effective swallow.[19] As children are dynamic, developing beings, the oral motor pattern may well change over time, particularly in the early years, before the child is 8 years old.[30,48]

Hypersensitivity requires implementation of an early desensitization programme.[48,49] For non-oral children, oral sensorimotor therapy can help to maintain oral motor movements, reduce hypersensitivity and may allow for better control of saliva and oral hygiene. It should be very carefully managed however, as oral stimulation may create greater production of saliva, which the child may not be able to control, thus increasing the risk of aspiration of secretions. Together with adapted and planned feeding techniques, oral sensorimotor therapy, if used frequently and consistently, can reduce oral defensiveness and improve the opportunities for better eating and drinking. It is only likely to be effective if carried out in a number of therapeutic sessions a day.[48]

Fatigue

As fatigue has such a marked effect on oral motor skills and swallow function, any feeding plan should include ways to reduce fatigue. This may mean shorter mealtimes but more frequent opportunities to eat, or more careful timing of meals throughout the day. The dietitian's expertise will be essential for this to be effective.

Behaviour

The clinician needs to consider behavioural issues as refusal of food means that any feeding plan cannot be implemented. Looking at causes is the first step. Consistencies of approach and good evidence-based strategies are needed.

Communication

Fundamental to the management of the whole eating and drinking process is the development of good communication between the child and the helper. The child should not be passive in the relationship; interactive and timely communications are important for effective management.[22] The training of parents and carers who feed a child is crucial in enskilling them to make accurate observations of signs of aspiration, of appropriate timing of each mouthful, of watching for likes and dislikes, pain or discomfort. Equally, good communication between members of the multidisciplinary team when setting goals will ensure a more cohesive feeding plan. Parents report that indecision and lack of agreement between professionals causes further distress and anxiety.[35]

Drooling

It has been estimated that significant drooling persists in up to 38% individuals with cerebral palsy.[50,51] It can have a detrimental effect on both the individual child and the family. Caregivers reported in Van der Burg's study that managing drooling was demanding in terms of changes of clothing, damage to communication devices, wiping chins, washing and coping with the social impact and effect on self-esteem.[52] Studies have shown that drooling is not a result of excessive saliva production but rather a combination of poor oral motor skills, inefficient and reduced swallowing and possible decreased sensory perception.[50,53] The factors that affect drooling are important in determining which treatment methods are most appropriate. But in all cases, a joint approach will be necessary. In most treatment options, a varied level of success has been reported, particularly in the long term.

A pharmacological approach has been used for some time with varying degrees of success. Anticholinergic drugs such as hyoscine and glycopyrronium bromide have been shown to reduce salivary flow effectively but side effects are common. However, they are used widely clinically and seem to decrease the need for wiping and changing of bibs etc.[52]

Botulinum toxin injections are increasingly reported to have a good effect on production of saliva with no side effects and high response rates up to a period of 24 weeks.[54] There needs to be further follow-up of these children to measure success over the long term.

Surgery for submandibular duct transposition is clearly invasive, can adversely affect the swallow and there are doubts about the long-term effectiveness of the treatment, but it has lead to some improvement in some individuals.[55] Intra-oral devices such as the Innsbruck Sensorimotor Activator and Regulator (ISMAR) have shown improvement in management of saliva and eating and drinking skills.[56] It appears to be a valid option for intervention. Again, longer term outcomes should be investigated. Training devices and behaviour modification have all been used to attempt to reduce drooling. Head control and position of the body have an important part to play in drooling management.

Oral motor therapy equally has shown some effect but longer term management remains a challenge. A practical suggestion is to use pressured dabbing, rather than wiping the mouth, to reduce confusing sensory input and help produce some lip closure. Oral hygiene should always be investigated as part of the assessment and intervention plan for drooling.

In summary, drooling needs careful consideration of all possible approaches by the multidisciplinary team, along with discussion with families about the expected outcomes for each child.

Summary

Eating and drinking are often impaired in the child with a neurodevelopmental disability. A multidisciplinary approach is needed in order to achieve safe and effective intake. The SLT can offer specialized assessment and therapeutic intervention for children and the family as part of the team in order to support and improve the day to day management of oral motor skills and swallowing. In some cases, oral feeding will not be safe or it will not meet the child's nutrition and hydration needs. Non-oral feeding will need to be considered. The discussion and process of introducing non-oral feeding should be undertaken honestly and sensitively with parents as part of the team. Only through the closest collaboration between the parents, SLT, dietitian, paediatrician and the rest of the team can we maximize nutrition and hydration and keep the child as safe as possible.

References

1. Fung EB, Samson-Fang L, Stallings VA et al. Feeding dysfunction is associated with poor growth and health status in children with cerebral palsy. *J Am Diet Assoc* 2002; **102**: 3–73.
2. Schwarz SM, Corredor J, Fisher-Medina J, Cohen J, Rabinowitz S. Diagnosis and treatment of feeding disorders in children with developmental disabilities. *Pediatrics* 2001; **108**: 671–6.
3. Griggs CA, Jones PM, Lee RE. Videofluoroscopic investigation of feeding disorders of children with multiple handicap. *Dev Med Child Neurol* 1989; **31**: 303–8.
4. Merritt PL, Riski JE, Glascott J, Johnson V. Videofluoroscopic Assessment of dysphagia in children with severe spastic cerebral palsy. *Dysphagia* 1994; **9**: 174–9.
5. Motion S, Northstone K, Emond A, Stucke S, Golding J. Early feeding problems in children with cerebral palsy: weight and neurodevelopmental outcomes. *Dev Med Child Neurol* 2002; **44**: 40–3.
6. Loughlin GM. Respiratory consequences of dysfunctional swallowing and aspiration. *Dysphagia* 1989; **3**: 126–30.
7. Couriel JM, Bisset R, Miller R, Thomas A, Clarke M. Assessment of feeding problems in neurodevelopmental handicap: a team approach. *Arch Dis Child* 1993; **69**: 609–13.
8. Royal College of Speech and Language Therapists (RCSLT). *RCSLT Clinical Guidelines*. Bicester: Speechmark Publishing, 2005.
9. Royal College of Speech and Language Therapists. *Communicating Quality*, 3rd edn. London: RCSLT, 2006.
10. Sullivan PB, Lambert B, Rose M, Ford-Adams M, Johnson A, Griffiths P. Prevalence and severity of feeding and nutritional problems in children with neurological impairment: Oxford Feeding Study. *Dev Med Child Neurol* 2000; **42**: 10–80.
11. Redstone F, West JF. The importance of postural control for feeding. *Pediatr Nurs* 2004; **30**: 97–100.
12. Strauss D, Ashwal S, Shavelle R, Eyman RK. Prognosis for survival and improvement in function in children with severe developmental disabilities. *J Pediatr* 1997; **131**: 712–17.
13. Morton R, Minford J, Ellis R, Pinnington L. Aspiration with dysphagia: the interaction between oropharyngeal and respiratory impairments. *Dysphagia* 2002; **17**: 192–6.
14. Reilly S, Skuse D, Mathisen B, Wolke D. The objective rating of oral-motor functions during feeding. *Dysphagia* 1995; **10**: 177–91.

15. Selley WG, Flack FC, Ellis RE, Brooks WA. The Exeter dysphagia assessment technique. *Dysphagia* 1990; **4**: 227–35.
16. Kenny DJ, Koheil RM, Greenberg J et al. Development of a multidisciplinary feeding profile for children who are dependent feeders. *Dysphagia* 1989; **4**: 16–28.
17. Morris SE. Development of oral-motor skills in the neurologically impaired child receiving non-oral feedings. *Dysphagia* 1989; **3**: 135–54.
18. Pelegano JP, Goepferd S, Bermel S. Mandibular range of motion in spastic quadraplegia. *Dev Med Child Neurol* 1992; **34**: 36.
19. Winstock A. *Eating and Drinking Difficulties in Children. A Guide for Practitioners.* Bicester: Speechmark Publishing, 2005.
20. Evans-Morris S, Dunn-Klien M. *Pre-Feeding Skills*, 2nd edn. San Antonio, TX: Therapy Skill Builders, 2000.
21. Bosma JF. Development of feeding. *Clin Nutr* 1986; **5**: 210–18.
22. Arvedson J, Brodsky L. *Pedaitric Swallowing and Feeding.* Albany: Singular Publishing Group, 2002.
23. McCurtin A. *The Manual of Paediatric Feeding Practice.* Oxon: Winslow Press, 1997.
24. Cass H, Wallis C, Ryan M, Reilly S, McHugh K. Assessing pulmonary consequences of dysphagia in children with neurological disabilities: when to intervene? *Dev Med Child Neurol* 2005; **47**: 347–52.
25. Heine RG, Reddihough DS, Catto-Smith AG. Gastro-oesophageal reflux and feeding problems after gastrostomy in children with severe neurological impairment. *Dev Med Child Neurol* 1995; **37**: 320–9.
26. Sullivan PB, Juszczak E, Lambert BR, Rose M, Ford-Adams ME, Johnson A. Impact of feeding problems on nutritional intake and growth: Oxford Feeding Study II. *Dev Med Child Neurol* 2002; **44**: 461–7.
27. DeMatteo C, Matovich D, Hjartarson A. Comparison of clinical and videofluoroscopic evaluation of children with feeding and swallowing difficulties. *Dev Med Child Neurol* 2005; **47**: 149–57.
28. Arvedson J, Rogers B, Buck G, Smart P, Msall M. Silent aspiration prominent in children with dysphagia. *Int J Pediatr Otorhinolaryngol* 1994; **28**: 173–81.
29. Siebens AA, Linden P. Dynamic imaging for swallowing reeducation. *Gastrointest Radiol* 1985; **10**: 251–3.
30. Arvedson J, Lefton-Greif M. *Pediatric Videofluoroscopic Swallow Studies: A Professional Manual with Caregivers Guidelines.* San Antonio, Tx: Communication Skill Builders, 1998.
31. Samson-Fang L, Butler C, O'Donnell M. Effects of gastrostomy feeding in children with cerebral palsy: an AACPDM evidence report. *Dev Med Child Neurol* 2003; **45**: 415–26.
32. Helfrich-Miller KR, Rector KL, Straka JA. Dysphagia: its treatment in the profoundly retarded patient with cerebral palsy. *Arch Phys Med Rehabil* 1986; **67**: 520–5.
33. Lee J, Blain S, Casas M, Kenny D, Berall G, Chau T. A radial basis classifier for the automatic detection of aspiration in children with dysphagia. *J Neuroengineering Rehabil* 2006; **3**: 14.
34. Rogers B, Arvedson J, Buck G, Smart P, Msall M. Characteristics of dysphagia in children with cerebral palsy. *Dysphagia* 1994; **9**: 69–73.
35. Townsley R, Robinson C. *Food for Thought.* Bristol: Nora Fry Research Centre, 2000.
36. Sullivan PB. Gastrointestinal problems in the neurologically impaired child. *Baillieres Clin Gastroenterol* 1997; **11**: 529–46.
37. Chatoor I, Schaefer S, Dickson L, Egan J. Non-organic failure to thrive: a developmental perspective. *Pediatr Ann* 1984; **13**: 829–35, 838, 840–2.
38. Mathison B, Worrall L, Masel J, Wall C, Shepherd RW. Feeding problems in infants with gastro-oesophageal reflux disease: a controlled study. *J Paediatr Child Health* 1999; **35**: 163–9.
39. Hawdon J, Beauregard N, Slattery J, Kennedy G. Identification of neonates at risk of developing feeding problems in infancy. *Dev Med Child Neurol* 2000; **42**: 235–9.
40. Satter E. Feeding dynamics: helping children to eat well. *J Pediatr Health Care* 1995; **9**: 178–84.
41. Peterson M, Kedia S, Davis P, Newman L, Temple C. Eating and feeding are not the same: caregivers' perceptions of gastrostomy feeding for children with cerebral palsy. *Dev Med Child Neurol* 2006; **48**: 713–17

42. Larnert G, Ekberg O. Positioning improves the oral and pharyngeal swallowing function in children with cerebral palsy. *Acta Paediatr* 1995; **84**: 689–92.
43. Cockerill H. *A Guide to Food Textures*. Speech and Language Special Interest Group in Paediatric Dysphagia, 2001. (Available from Helen Cockerill, Consultant SLT, Newcomen Centre, Guy's Hospital, Thomas Street, London, SE1 9RT.)
44. Morton RE, Wheatley R, Minford J. Respiratory tract infections due to direct and reflux aspiration in children with severe neurodisability. *Dev Med Child Neurol* 1999; **41**: 329–34.
45. Rempel G, Moussavi Z. The effect of viscosity on the breath-swallow pattern of young people with cerebral palsy. *Dysphagia* 2005; **20**: 108–12.
46. Sullivan PB, Rosenbloom L. *Feeding the Disabled Child*. London: MacKeith Press, 1996.
47. Pinnington L. Effects of consistent food presentation on oral-motor skill acquisition in children with severe neurological impairment. *Dysphagia* 2000; **15**: 213–23.
48. Manno C, Fox C, Eicher P, Kerwin M. Early oral-motor interventions for pediatric feeding problems: what, when and how. *J Early Intensive Behaviour Intervention* 2005; **2**: 145–54.
49. Rommel N, De Meyer AM, Feenstra L, Veereman-Wauters G. The complexity of feeding problems in 700 infants and young children presenting to a tertiary care institution *J Pediatr Gastroenterol Nutr* 2003; **37**: 75–84.
50. Senner JE, Logemann J, Zecker S, Gaebler-Spira D. Drooling, saliva production, and swallowing in cerebral palsy. *Dev Med Child Neurol* 2004; **46**: 801–6.
51. Blasco PA. Management of drooling: 10 years after the Consortium on Drooling, 1990. *Dev Med Child Neurol* 2002; **44**: 778–81.
52. van der Burg JJ, Jongerius PH, van HK, van LJ, Rotteveel JJ. Drooling in children with cerebral palsy: effect of salivary flow reduction on daily life and care. *Dev Med Child Neurol* 2006; **48**: 103–7.
53. Sochaniwskyj AE, Koheil RM, Bablich K, Milner M, Kenny DJ. Oral motor functioning, frequency of swallowing and drooling in normal children and in children with cerebral palsy. *Arch Phys Med Rehabil* 1986; **67**: 866–74.
54. Jongerius PH, van den Hoogen FJ, van LJ, Gabreels FJ, van HK, Rotteveel JJ. Effect of botulinum toxin in the treatment of drooling: a controlled clinical trial. *Pediatrics* 2004; **114**: 620–7.
55. Uppal HS, De R, D'Souza AR, Pearman K, Proops DW. Bilateral submandibular duct relocation for drooling: an evaluation of results for the Birmingham Children's Hospital. *Eur Arch Otorhinolaryngol* 2003; **260**: 48–51.
56. Scott A, Johnson H. *A Practical Approach to the Management of Saliva Control*, 2nd edn. Austin, TX: Pro-Ed, 2004.

Chapter 4

Feeding and Dietetic Assessment and Management

Bridget R Lambert and Wee Meng Han

The development of feeding skills

The individual feeding ability and skills of a child overwhelmingly influence whether or not they are able to ingest an appropriate dietary intake sufficient to sustain their nutritional status, growth and overall development.[1-3]

Children unaffected by neurological impairment can be expected to learn to eat and feed themselves competently by school age, that is, when they are about 5 years old. For the child with disabilities, however, the normal anticipated progression and acquisition of independent self-feeding skills may never be realized, or only up to a certain stage. Nevertheless, as food is such a basic and vital human requirement, all children, unless it is contraindicated as a result of an unsafe swallow and risk of aspiration, should be given the opportunity to learn to eat and feed themselves, and enjoy their food, even though for some this presents more of a challenge than for others. In this section, the development of feeding skills in children without neurological impairment is described. This information can be used to determine what level a child with disabilities may have achieved and what might be the next stage in this process that they can reach or be encouraged to progress towards. Consideration can then be given to what can be done practically to enable and promote more successful and proficient feeding, and achieve a child's individual potential in this important area of normal, everyday life.

Development of eating and drinking skills in children

Being able to feed successfully depends on the interactions of many nerves, muscles and reflexes. Whereas we take it for granted, it is a complex function that requires practice and time to develop, from infancy through to early childhood.

- Eating and drinking involves the coordination of 31 pairs of muscles and 6 cranial nerves.

- The mouth, jaw, palate and tongue structures all need to be in place and function correctly.
- Teeth are important for the chewing, biting and grinding of food.
- The airway needs to be protected competently or aspiration occurs.
- Hand to mouth coordination must be possible if the person is to learn to feed independently.
- Positioning of the body in an upright position is also important.

Table 4.1 shows an example of the sequence of infant development and feeding skills.[4]

Infants
The developmental skills attained during the first year of life in terms of mouth movements and hand and body control are illustrated in Table 4.1 and it also details what the infant without neurological impairment can be expected to manage in terms of eating solids and drinking liquids. There in some overlap between stages, and babies develop at their own pace. Hence, ages at which skills are attained will vary, as will how successful an infant is at them. Additionally, infants require encouragement, interaction and opportunity from the person that is feeding them for each stage to be achieved and developed.

From birth until around 4–6 months of life, the infant is only capable of sucking and swallowing milk from the breast or a bottle. They need supporting while feeding as they have poor muscle control of the head, neck and trunk.

From the age of around 4–6 months, the infant's mouth movements and hand and body control become more sophisticated. They can move their jaws up and down and transfer food from different areas within the mouth. Muscle tone is stronger. The baby can sit upright with support and control its head. At this age, smooth, puréed foods, for example, ground rice, fruits and vegetables can be introduced. They can be controlled within the mouth and swallowed without choking.

Between 6 and 9 months, infants can hold objects in their hands and thus begin to finger feed. Some will have a few teeth. They can munch foods more confidently and cope with a more textured, lumpier and mashed up diet. If offered a spoon this will generally be accepted and grabbed. The infant wants to be in charge of feeding and may turn their head away when food is offered as if to say 'no! I want to do it myself!' Muscle tone improves and they can sit upright unsupported.

Between 8 and 11 months, tongue and lip and hand movements mature. Many infants develop the ability to drink from a cup. They become more competent at self-feeding using their hands. They can now manage chopped up soft foods. Feeding will be messy but fun. Touching and handling food is an important part of learning to self-feed and should be encouraged.

Table 4.1 Sequence of infant development and feeding skills[4]

Baby's approximate age	Developmental skills		
	Mouth patterns	Hand and body control	Baby can:
Birth to 5 months	Sucking/ swallowing reflex Tongue thrust reflex Poor lip closure	Poor control of head, neck, trunk	Swallow liquids but pushes most solid objects from the mouth
4–6 months	Draws in lower lip as spoon is removed from mouth Up and down movement Immediately transfers food from front to back of tongue to swallow	Sits with support Good head control Uses whole hand to grasp objects (palmar grasp)	Take in a spoonful of puréed or strained food and swallow it without choking Control the position of food in the mouth
5–9 months	Up and down munching movement Positions food between jaws for chewing	Begins to sit alone, unsupported Begins to use thumb and index finger to pick up objects (pincer grasp)	Begin to eat mashed foods Eat from a spoon easily
8–11 months	Complete side to side tongue movement Begins to curve lips around rim of cup	Sits alone easily	Begin to eat ground or finely chopped food Begin to feed self with hands Drink from a cup
10–11 months	Rotary chewing (grinding)	Begins to put spoon in mouth Begins to hold cup	Eat chopped food, small pieces of soft, cooked food

By their first birthday, the infant will have come a long way from total dependence to a degree of autonomy with self-feeding ability. They will have mastered the basics, be able to use a spoon and have the oral skill to manage a chopped up soft diet easily. They will however, still need some manual assistance and supervision to ensure they are feeding safely and achieving an adequate intake of food.

Toddlers
Between 1 and 3 years of age, children still need a degree of help and supervision from a carer with feeding, but like to do it themselves. Their independence with self-feeding and desire to do this grows and may lead to frustration if they can not do this just how they want, or they are not permitted to do it. Tempers may become frayed at mealtimes. Most children will need help with the cutting up or chopping of foods until about the age of 3 or 4 years. Some may have difficulty chewing foods such as meat, especially when cutting teeth.

Playing with food is an important part of learning about it; what it is, what it feels like, where it goes, what it tastes like. It is vital that children are allowed and encouraged to do this. Helping to choose foods for meals, going shopping, simple cooking and food preparation are all other aspects to be promoted within the context of normal feeding development.

Children in this age group begin to voice their opinions more and say what foods they like and don't like. The range of foods toddlers are willing to eat can be limited. This can cause great concern for parents, who get very anxious that their child is not eating a nutritionally adequate diet. Generally, for children who are thriving, energetic and healthy despite a self-restricted diet reassurance is all that is required as most grow out of this phase. Eating outside the home environment, for example at nursery, or with others – peers, non-parental relatives – can also be conducive to improved dietary intake.

Young children
Over the next few years, and almost certainly by around 5 years of age, children are able to feed themselves independently and need no help from a carer. They have a full set of teeth and can therefore tackle most textures and types of foods, although some foods such as apples with tough skins that require biting, or hard crusts, may prove too difficult to manage competently. The majority of the skills required to use utensils, (spoons, forks and finally knives), to manipulate them and coordinate their use are mastered, as the child develops further neuromuscular function and coordination.

Eating with others and observing their behaviour is important in helping to develop the social aspects of feeding. By this age, children have generally adopted their family's attitudes towards eating, have reasonably acceptable table manners, are able to sit at the table during a meal and join in the conversation. They are also now able to fully verbalize their needs, say when they are full, forage for food, make choices and be influenced about food by others, e.g. television, peers, older siblings. They are generally more accepting of the food given to them and are a lot less fussy. Food fads from earlier years tend to have been forgotten.

So, in conclusion, the infant without neurological impairment transforms from being totally dependant on others to feed them, to learning to self-feed with some assistance and input from a carer by the age of around 3, to being a young child feeding independently and competently with utensils, usually by the age of 5 years. They will have evolved from being fed by one other in isolation to sharing meals and eating with others. Their oral skills will have matured from being able only to suck and swallow milk to consuming a diet typical of their society with a full range of tastes and textures.

Eating and drinking skills in children with neurological impairment

Not all children with neurological impairment have feeding problems, or if they experience difficulties, have them to the extent where some form of intervention is required. The degree to which disability affects a child's feeding ability is very variable and individual.[5,6] Profoundly disabled children with very obvious feeding problems are generally totally reliant on another to feed them and need some form of intervention to ensure an adequate nutritional intake from food and fluids, be it modification to textures and consistencies through to the insertion of a gastrostomy. Regardless of disability level though, relatives can spend many hours each day preparing and giving food and drink to their child, and this can be an unpleasant, slow, messy and frustrating business.[7] Mealtimes can be prolonged and unpleasant as it takes longer and requires more effort to feed. Food and drink may be dropped or spilt because of difficulties with the use of hands, fingers, cutlery and utensils. Oral insufficiency may mean problems with biting, chewing and swallowing, resulting in coughing, spluttering and choking while eating and drinking. These problems may mean a child is fed on their own if eating habits are offensive and off putting to others, meaning the child is excluded from the social side of eating through no fault of their own. Many disabled children thus continue to be dependent on others throughout their lives for partial or total assistance with feeding and drinking, sometimes to save effort, energy and social embarrassment, even though they may be able to self-feed to some degree. The time they take to do this may just be too long to be tolerated within their daily schedules.

However, it is to be remembered that just as children without disability develop and increase in ability with age and maturity this can be the experience of children with disabilities. Depending on their individual cognitive and physical abilities they may continue to gain skills and learn, albeit at a different rate and to a different level of competence from their peer group without neurodevelopmental disabilities. Over a more extended time period they too may learn to feed themselves independently. Some that needed a lot of help and support as young children may go on to eventually require only minimum input from other people, therapists and gadgets, and manage consistencies and amounts of food previously thought entirely inappropriate for them.[8]

Carers' experiences of feeding children with neurological impairment

We know from research described in other chapters in this book that disabled children are frequently difficult and challenging to feed, and the problems include the special preparation of foods, the feeding itself and the clearing up afterwards.[9,10] Yet, what is it like to feed and care for a child who has feeding difficulties because of neurological impairment?

To provide some insight into feeding experiences among this group of children and their carers, we will consider some of the qualitative data collected (by the author, BL) as part of semi-structured interviews conducted during the Oxford Feeding Study an epidemiological investigation carried out within a defined geographical area of four counties in England.[11,12] The aim of the investigation was to estimate the prevalence and severity of feeding and nutritional problems in children with neurological impairment. The Oxford Register of Early Childhood Impairment was used to identify 377 children with motor deficit plus or minus feeding problems, who were sent a validated postal questionnaire on feeding and other issues such as general health, level of disability, services received and medications being taken. Of the 271 replies (return rate of 72%), 100 children, who exhibited a wide range of level of disability, from mild to moderate to severe, were randomly selected and visited at home.

At each home visit, as well as verifying the information filled in on the questionnaire, information on dietary intake was collected and nutritional status and growth measured anthropometrically. These results are not included in this section. During the home visit, parents and carers were asked about feeding their disabled child. The intention was to investigate if a degree of neurological impairment, mild and moderate or severe, had an impact on feeding ability and to try and find out more about the experience of feeding such children. A semi-structured interview, including questions such as those below, was used and the data obtained analysed quantitatively:

- the child's self-feeding ability;
- estimated time spent feeding each day by carer;
- types, textures of foods managed; specific problems with eating; foods and drinks preferred/enjoyed;
- were separate foods and meals prepared for the child from the rest of the family?
- where and with whom did the child eat?
- did the child make their needs and preferences for food and drink known, and how?
- did the child eat out in public, and if so, what was this experience like.

The 100 children visited in their homes comprised 40 girls and 60 boys, who ranged in age from 5–13 years, with a mean of 9.1 years. Ninety had some degree of cerebral palsy and ten had a variety of developmental and genetic problems resulting in neurological impairments. For the purposes of analysis, the 100 were divided into two groups based on walking ability and hence physical mobility. Those classified as mild and moderately physically disabled, 31 in total, were mobile. They could either walk independently, with or without the use of aids, such as a frame, special boots for support or help from another person. Those in the severely physically disabled group (69) were unable to walk at all and were dependent on a wheelchair to get around. Children in both groups had varying degrees of upper limb and hand function and cognitive ability.

The two groups contained a diverse assortment of intellectual abilities; some in the mild/moderate group were able to walk quite independently but had severe cognitive deficits. Others in this group were fully mobile and at mainstream school but had a hemi or diplegia with resultant difficulty in walking.

In the severe group, although all had a physical disability requiring the use of a wheelchair a few were in mainstream schools with age appropriate cognitive function; however, most were profoundly globally developmentally delayed.

Help required with feeding
With regard to self-feeding, 7/31 (23%) of children in the mild/moderate group were able to feed themselves although 24/31 (77%) sometimes required help from a carer at mealtimes. This help included the chopping up of certain foods, the loading of food onto a spoon so then the child could use it themselves to place food in their mouth or the actual feeding of the child. The help was given either partially during each meal, for example, towards the end as the child was tiring, or as required, therefore not necessarily at every meal. In the severely disabled group of 69 children only 1/69 (2%) required no assistance with feeding, 41/60 (59%) sometimes needed help and 27/69 (39%) always needed feeding by another person.

The mean age of the 100 children was 9.1 years (range 5–13 years). As stated earlier, most children without disability will require some degree of help with feeding up to the age of about 3–4 years, but by around 5 they can feed themselves. In comparison with children without disability, in this study two-thirds of children with a mild/ moderate disability and the majority 65/69 (94%) of those who were severely disabled were either totally reliant on another to feed them or needed a significant amount of assistance with feeding after the age of 5. This has obvious implications for carers in terms of the time involved and supervision required at meal times when the child is at an age where usually they would be expected to be able to manage for themselves.

Swallowing and eating difficulty
To assess swallowing and feeding difficulty, as described by the parent or carer, the four-point scale derived by Reilly et al in 1996 was used for comparison.[1] This divides swallowing and feeding ability, and the types of foods and liquids able to be managed by the child into four levels.

1. Has no feeding problems, manages a normal diet.
2. Mild difficulty, manages chopped or mashed foods.
3. Moderate difficulty, requires well-mashed, chopped and moist foods.
4. Severe difficulty, manages thickened fluids, purées or needs tube feeds.

The group of children with a mild or moderate disability had few problems with eating, and apart from 2/31 (6%), all were able to eat a normal textured diet with a minimum of modification required (levels 1 and 2). However, in the severely disabled group, although half had moderate and serious problems with eating and required major modifications to texture and presentation (levels 3 and 4), the other half were able to eat a normal diet, or required minimum modification to their food (levels 1 and 2). One reason for this was that many carers, particularly of the older severely disabled children in this group reported that even though their child had problems with eating, their abilities had improved with age and practice. Input regarding feeding from health professionals -speech therapists, occupational therapists and physiotherapists – was mentioned as being of significant help in this regard. Thus, even though the common perception is that being severely disabled means feeding problems and eating difficulties for life, there is potential for improvement for some. Some parents reported their children were determined to eat foods not usually of a suitable texture and consistency for them to competently manage (e.g. pizza, sausages), either because they liked and enjoyed them, or wanted to join in with what other people were having at mealtimes.

Duration of feeding times

The Oxford Feeding Study and others have noted that the parents of some disabled children spend many hours each day feeding their children. This is because of a slow pace of eating and inability to chew and swallow food competently.[13,14]

An estimate of the time spent eating food orally by each of the 100 children in the study was requested. This included any time spent feeding orally by carers. It is acknowledged that as it was an estimate of time taken there is likely to be some inaccuracy. For some profoundly disabled children fed orally, the feeding process described (and observed) was unpleasant and prolonged, hence the carer may have overestimated the duration of daily feedings as it might have seemed that was all they did all day.

The average time spent eating by a young child without disability is around 1 hour a day. In this sample, although about half, 14/31 (45%), of those mildly and moderately disabled ate their food orally within this timeframe, the rest took up to 2 hours daily. No-one took longer.

In the severely disabled group, although one-third, 24/69 (35%), took between 3 and 6 hours daily to be fed orally, 36/69 (52%) managed to eat and or be fed in 2 hours per day or less. In this group 9/69 (13%) were tube fed.

In both disability groups oral feeding times longer than the norm of 1 hour each day were experienced, with again, implications for the lives of these children and their carers.

Self-feeding abilities and feeding practices

Carers were asked to describe their child's self-feeding skills. In the mild and moderately disabled group, all 31 were able to finger feed i.e. pick up pieces of solid food using their fingers, such as a biscuit or slice of fruit, and put it into their mouths. 23/31 (74%) had the manual dexterity to use ordinary spoons and forks (but not knives) to eat with.

8/31 (26%) used specially adapted cutlery and utensils. All 31 sat at a table at mealtimes; a few required special seating for support. However, 3/31 (10%) sadly always ate by themselves as a result of behavioural problems at mealtimes, and 6/31 (19%) had meals prepared separately for them from the rest of the family because of different texture requirements.

In the severely disabled group, 29/69 (42%) were able to finger feed themselves to some degree yet still required significant help from someone. In this group 35/69 (51%) always had different meals prepared for them from the rest of the family because they needed food of a different texture. Over a half, 37/69 (54%), were always given their meals by themselves; they never ate in company apart from the person who was feeding them being present. Often this was for valid reasons, such as it was too disruptive for the other family members; it took a long time so the meal of the person feeding them would get cold; the child coughed, spluttered and choked excessively or there were behavioural issues. For the feeder (the majority of feeders in this study were mothers), it was described as an isolating experience; being shut in another room, often for long periods of time. Feeding a difficult child is not pleasant, and many reported that they did not like this aspect of caring for their child at all. It was considered necessary but very unrewarding.

Some of the negative comments by carers that were recorded during interview were as follows.

- 'Feeding is time consuming and messy.'
- 'Feeding my child means I have no time for myself or the rest of the family.'
- 'I feel like I'm always feeding him.'
- 'I get fed up feeding, it's boring.'
- 'I'm the only one in the family who can feed my child.'
- 'I get no help with feeding her.'

Yet, some comments were positive such as those that follow.

- 'It's my way of caring for my child.'
- 'Feeding is all I can do for him – I can't play with him like his brother.'
- 'Feeding my child is very important to me.'
- 'Although she doesn't eat nicely, it's important to me that we include her in family mealtimes.'

The comments above reveal that the feeding of a child by their carer encompasses many complex physical, emotional and social processes aside from its basic purpose of providing nourishment. At its best it is a very meaningful activity, particularly in terms of facilitating a bond or relationship between the child and its caregivers. Having a child that is rewarding to feed and responds positively and appropriately when being fed is obviously of mutual benefit. Unfortunately, this is not usually the experience of the carers of disabled children dependent on them for their nourishment. The positive intimate interaction there can be between the two, between the feeder and the fed, does not take place or exist.

Disabled children tend to have a lot of specialized equipment taking up room and space in the home. Adapted seating for eating in or special attachments for wheelchairs such as trays was present for 100% of the severely neurologically impaired group visited in this study. However, these were not always used and some children were fed in their carer's arms, regardless of appropriateness or safety.

Eating out socially
Of the mild and moderately disabled children 25/31 (81%) enjoyed meals out socially on a regular basis with their families, either in a public place such as a restaurant or in other people's homes. However, some carers said that because of their child's problems, this would attract unwanted public attention. This was the reason why the remaining 6/31 (19%) didn't eat out with their child as they found it was all too difficult and embarrassing.

In comparison, in the severely disabled group, 53/69 (77%) had regular trips out with their families to eat in restaurants and other peoples homes. The remainder (17/69, 24%) never took their child out to eat in public, describing it as too traumatic, as they experienced too much unwelcome attention regarding their child's disability and eating problems to feel comfortable with it. In addition, the wheelchair could be a big problem in terms of getting into and accessing places. It was easier to stay at home.

This illustrates that feeding problems for disabled children are socially excluding, both within the family and in wider society. Obviously some children, because of their profound disabilities, are unaware of what is going on around them and it is the carers who chose to tolerate or not the problems this creates. However, some carers reported that their children (generally the older ones in this sample) were aware for themselves of the difficulties it generated when they did eat in public and were embarrassed about eating outside their own home environment. Some children preferred to eat alone or in select company to avoid making others feel uncomfortable while they were eating. Interestingly, some carers stated that although feeding their disabled child outside the home might be troubling for members of the public, they were still determined to carry on taking their child out to eat as they saw it as a very important aspect of their social lives and nothing to be ashamed of.

Children's food preferences – likes and dislikes
These turned out to be not that different from the general child population in both disability groups. Chips, roast dinners, chocolate, pasta and cakes were mentioned as regularly preferred foods based on taste alone. Milk, fruit juice, fizzy drinks and tea were favourite drinks. Fruit and vegetables were not popular.

Foods reported as being difficult to eat
For those disabled children without profound eating and feeding difficulties, some foods were described as being more challenging to eat. Meats, such as beef and pork, were reported as being too chewy for some; crusts on bread would be removed and left on the plate as they were too hard; some children were adverse to lumps in foods and others wouldn't eat hard foods needing to be bitten into e.g. apples, pears. However, this list is not untypical of the sorts of foods avoided by many children without disabilities and adults. Some parents reported that their child, despite oral motor difficulties, would eat a favourite food even if it was of an unsuitable texture.

Indication by the child of hunger and thirst
One of the common issues reported by parents during interviews was interpreting what their child needed, especially for those children with absent or poor communication skills. How do you tell if a child that doesn't speak is hungry, thirsty, and full or doesn't like what you are giving them? Many said they had to rely on the body language of their child or just guess. Of the carers of the mild and moderately disabled children 24/31 (77%) said they were able to ask their child these questions and obtain a verbal response from them. However, as some children had cognitive impairment, the interaction might not always be meaningful. Of this group 7/31 (24%) could not verbalize but could use some form of gesturing or behaviour to indicate their needs.

Communication problems regarding hunger and thirst were, not surprisingly, greatest in the severely disabled group. In this group 29/69 (42%) had no communication skills and were thus unable to indicate to their carers if they wanted food or drink or had had enough. Thirty-five per cent (24/69) used some form of behaviour or body language to indicate what they might want and 16/69 (23%) could verbalize their needs, but as with the mild and moderate group, cognitive impairment often meant that the child's messages were misunderstood.

Interestingly, it seemed that many carers were keen to involve their child in choosing what they would like to eat or drink. All the parents and carers of children in the mild and moderately disabled group (100%) and 23/69 (34%) in the severely disabled group said that their children were able to make such choices, but whether this was a true, conscious choice all the time they often could not be certain. However, children can communicate in very subtle ways to their carers, ways in which someone not familiar with the child would be unable to discern. It could be carers can interpret some requests from their child that a stranger could not.

Eating and self-feeding are complex processes that normally are learnt within the first 5–6 years of life. Children with neurological disabilities often struggle to feed competently, and the development of their eating and feeding skills can be delayed. Severely disabled children tend to have the worst feeding problems, but even those with mild and moderate neurological impairments may struggle and need assistance with feeding for longer than their peers without disability. For carers, feeding a disabled child can be tiring, frustrating, socially limiting, messy and time consuming, yet they may regard feeding as something positive they can do for their child. Given time, practise and appropriate input, some disabled children can progress with their self-feeding skills as they get older, meaning they are then not reliant on others to feed them.

Dietetic assessment of nutritional intake

Dietitians working with children with neurological impairment will use the information gained from an assessment of nutritional intake to either provide reassurance that the child is receiving an appropriate diet or use it to recommend ways of improving it. Acquiring precise detail on exactly what a child is consuming and how they achieve it can be difficult. There are many problems in obtaining reliable information on food intake. Overestimation of the food and fluid intake of an individual, using food diaries, dietary recall and food frequency questionnaires is known to have inherent inaccuracies and difficulties.[15] This has been noted as an issue by researchers investigating the dietary intakes of children with neurological impairment, for example, Stallings et al,[16] Fung et al[2] and Sullivan et al.[17]

However, this process will be very worthwhile. It will make any dietary advice given to parents and carers more practical and hopefully more readily implemented, and ultimately help improve nutritional status, general health and well-being. The British Dietetic Association Specialist Paediatric Group has produced a professional consensus statement to address the issue of the dietetic assessment of children with neurological impairment. This document endorses this as being a good and important professional practice for dietitians to carry out when involved in the care of such individuals.[18]

It is not just the foods and drinks they have orally but other factors such as meal patterns, types of foods able to be eaten, mealtime environment, self-feeding ability, behaviour, duration of meals and types of equipment required that are additional pieces of information that are all useful for the dietitian who is assessing a child. Appendix 6 has an example form that can be used as a guide for obtaining an overview of both feeding and dietary intake.

Prior to seeing a child for the first time, it is helpful, to both the carer and dietitian, if a 3-day food diary be completed and brought along to the consultation. Two weekdays and a weekend day will generally give a reasonable representation of normal intake. The diary will act as a source of useful information during the consultation and as a prompt and reminder of what the child usually manages. The child's carer should record in as much detail as possible everything that the child actually eats and drinks during the period of recording. To gain an idea of portion sizes, the use of household measures (such as 'a slice of', 'a tablespoon of') or the weight of the food in a packet or carton if this is available, should be noted. Items consumed outside the home, for example, at school or in other people's houses, need to be recorded, as well as details such as the timing of meals and their duration, consistency of foods given and brand names of products. Although food records, recall (diet history) and food frequency questionnaires are not 100% accurate in obtaining reliable information when assessing the dietary intakes of children with neurological impairment, nonetheless they are helpful tools for assessing meal patterns and the types of food offered and eaten. They can at least provide information in respect of food groups consumed.

Observation by the dietitian of the child during a meal is immensely useful. It can provide insight into details such as the interaction between the child and feeder, the pace of feeding, losses of food and fluid from the mouth and how this is dealt with (scooped up and replaced or removed?), the environment feeding takes place in and the position of the child and feeder during mealtimes. This is information that a carer may find difficult to describe and is therefore best witnessed by the health care professional.

Ideally, a feeding observation should be done in the child's home or other familiar location, such as school or nursery, where he or she is usually fed. Alternatively, parents or carers may be willing to film or video a mealtime at home so there are no distractions from being in a strange location or having other people present. The child's usual feeder should be the one to give the meal. The involvement of other multidisciplinary team members, such as the occupational therapist or speech and language therapist can be invaluable in terms of provision of a more holistic approach to assessing dietary intake and provision and institution of improvements in feeding as appropriate. Feeding observation should be used as a regular method of continued assessment and monitoring once any dietary recommendations have been made.

Once an estimate of food intake has been obtained, a computer software package such as 'Diet Plan' (Forestfield Software) can be used for analysis. Depending on the types of foods eaten, certain nutrients may be under- or overconsumed compared with recommended daily intakes, such as the UK Dietary Reference Values (DRVs) (1991).[19] For example, children requiring a diet that is puréed and very smooth may have a high intake of calcium if dairy foods predominate, such as yoghurts, custard, oat cereal made up with milk, and milk itself. Fibre and iron intakes may be low, as may vitamin C and folate intakes, as certain foods may not be readily eaten or offered due to their taste or texture.[17] A child who has feeding difficulties necessitating food modification and over reliance on one particular food group is at risk of micronutrient deficiencies. Dietary advice should be given to ensure a balanced diet is being offered to the child, supplemented with particular foods or prescribable vitamins, minerals or trace elements added in if necessary. This is explored in more detail later on in this chapter.

Energy and nutrient requirements

Providing optimal nutrition for children with neurodevelopment disabilities is a challenge. Fundamental to ensuring optimal nutrition is the specification of an adequate energy intake. Several studies have investigated the body composition and the energy expenditure in children with neurological impairment.[16,20,21] Bandini et al found that the fat-free mass, resting metabolic rate and total energy expenditure were significantly lower in the nine adolescents with cerebral palsy and the nine with myelodysplasia than the control group they studied.[20] The differences observed in the relationship between fat-free mass and resting metabolic rate between the cerebral palsy and myelodysplasia group suggested that the type of paralysis may affect basal energy expenditure. Stallings et al measured the energy expenditure pattern in a group of adolescents with spastic quadriplegic cerebral palsy.[16] In concurrence with the findings from Bandini et al[20] the total energy expenditure of children with spastic quadriplegic cerebral palsy was found to be significantly lower than that of the control group. Thus, the suggestion that the mechanical inefficiency of poorly controlled, volitional movement characteristic of spastic quadriplegic cerebral palsy creates an extraordinary high energy expenditure was not supported by the results of the study. In addition, the resting energy expenditure adjusted for fat-free mass was lower in the poorly nourished than in the adequately nourished group of children, implying an ability to adapt metabolically to the poorly nourished condition. A decade later, Sullivan et al also demonstrated that that the fat-free mass of children with spastic quadriplegic cerebral palsy was significantly lower than that of the reference population of age- and sex-matched children.[22] Further comparison showed that the gastrostomy-fed group had on average higher fat mass than the orally-fed group.[18] Although the difference was not statistically significant, it highlighted a potential for overfeeding these children with disabilities, particularly among those who are artificially fed. It is, therefore, clear from these studies that the energy recommendations for healthy populations or the energy requirements estimated from standard equations may not be applicable in this population where there are alterations in body composition and physical activity level.

There is a variety of approaches to estimate the energy needs of children with neurological impairment, such as those based on the recommended nutrient intakes (or recommended daily allowances) for chronological age, or adjusted for height, as well as those based on an estimated basal energy expenditure or basal energy expenditure adjusted for other factors, such as activity level.[23] Short stature occurs commonly among children with moderate to profound learning disability; therefore, using length, not weight, to estimate the energy needs had been proposed by Culley and Middleton,[24] as well as being supported by Bandini et al.[21] Krick et al proposed a complicated formula based on the basal metabolic rate, adjusted for muscle tone, ambulation and additional growth factor for catch-up growth where appropriate.[23] The 'Krick' formula was validated in 30 inpatients, and found to be a more potent predictor of energy requirements than the recommended daily allowance method.[23] Marchand and Motil reported that children with spastic quadriplegic cerebral palsy may grow normally with energy as low as 61 ± 15% of the recommended daily intake for age and sex; thus the resting energy expenditure calculated using standard equations, multiplied by a factor of 1.1 (instead of 1.5–1.6 in healthy children) may be sufficient.[25] Box 4.1 summarizes the methods currently used to determine dietary energy requirements in children with neurological impairment.[25]

Current dietetic consensus opinion in the UK is to use height age as a basis to estimate energy needs, as it is known that children with neurodeveopmental disability are smaller than their non-disabled counterparts, with adjustment depending on weight goals.[26] However, in practice, Almond et al[26] suggested that the energy requirement is often no more than 75% of the estimated average requirements, which are estimates of energy intakes for the free-living healthy population for height age and is often considerably less.

Box 4.1 Methods to determine dietary energy requirements in children with neurological impairment[25]

Dietary reference intake standards for basal energy expenditure(BEE)
Energy intake (kcal/d) = BEE × 1.1, where BEE is calculated as:

Male 66.5 + (13.75 × weight in kg) + (5.003 × height in cm) – (6.775 × age)
Female 665.1 + (9.56 × weight in kg) + (1.850 × height in cm) – (4.676 × age)

Indirect calorimetry[23]
Energy intake (kcal/d) = [basal energy expenditure (BMR) × muscle tone × activity] + growth, where:

BMR (kcal/d) = body surface area (m^2) × standard metabolic rate (kcal/m^2/h) × 24h
Muscle tone = 0.9 if decreased, 1.0 if normal, and 1.1 if increased
Activity = 1.1 if bedridden, 1.2 if wheelchair dependent or crawling, and 1.3 if ambulatory
Growth – 5 kcal/g of desired weight gain (normal and catch-up growth)

Height[24]
15 kcal/cm in children without motor dysfunction
14 kcal/cm in children with motor dysfunction who are ambulatory
11 kcal/cm in children who are non-ambulatory

Nevertheless, any method used to predict energy needs must be viewed as a preliminary guide and there must be close observation and modification of the nutritional programme, based on the needs of the individual child, to ensure proper linear and somatic growth.[19] This process is likely to require an extended period of monitoring of weight and intake, with subsequent adjustment of energy intake periodically in response to weight changes until an optimal intake for the desired weight goal is achieved.[21]

When the dietary energy is modified to meet the desired growth rate, it is essential to ensure provision of adequate protein and micronutrients in the diet.[25] A case report of a child with spastic quadriplegic cerebral palsy on gastrostomy feeding since the age of 2 years illustrated the importance of evaluating the nutrient density on low calorie diets.[27] At 11 years of age, despite a calorie intake slightly above her basal metabolic rate, she was found to be in negative nitrogen balance. An increase of calories and protein for a month restored positive nitrogen balance, while her body weight and renal function remained stable.

In the absence of evidence-based nutrient recommendations for children with neurological impairment, the recommendations for protein, vitamins and minerals for healthy children in the local population is suggested.[25] It is assumed that children with uncomplicated cerebral palsy have vitamin and mineral requirements comparable with those of typically developing children.[27]

Dietary reference values (DRVs)[19] are estimates of the amounts of energy and nutrients needed by different populations in the UK, and comprise three estimates:

- the estimated average requirements (EAR);
- the reference nutrient intakes (RNI); and
- the lower reference nutrient intakes (LRNI).

The EAR is an estimate of the mean requirement, i.e. approximately 50% of the population will require less, and the other 50% will require more. The RNI estimates the amount of nutrient that will ensure that the needs of nearly all (97.5%) of the population are being met, whereas the LRNI is the amount of nutrient that will only be sufficient for a small number (2.5%) of the population. The DRVs are useful recommendations; however, it should be remembered that the DRVs were devised for populations. Thus, for practical purpose in individuals, aiming for intakes between the RNI and the LRNI would usually be acceptable.

Dietary reference intakes (DRIs)[28] are the equivalent of the DRVs in the United States and have been more recently updated there than the UK. In addition, some nutrients also have established upper tolerable intake levels, which is the maximum level of daily nutrient that is likely to pose no risk of adverse effects.

Fluid requirements

Fluid requirements of children with neurological impairment may not be different from those without neurological impairment. However, a child who receives his/her nutrition solely from milk feeds will be expected to have a higher fluid requirement than another child who is eating a mixed diet. In the first instance, fluid requirements are typically calculated based on body weight (Table 4.2). In the second instance, it is based on the age and weight so that the fluid requirements can be calculated. It has been found that 600–900 ml per day is generally sufficient, although it may be higher in hot weather and the DRV (Table 4.3) provides a guideline.[29] Physical signs are important to determine whether a child is hydrated sufficiently. The signs of insufficient hydration include: strong-smelling nappies, yellow urine, fewer wet nappies than the norm (typically 6 to 8 in infants, 4 to 5 in older children), dry lips and skin, episodes of urinary tract infection and finally constipation. Meeting the fluid requirements can be difficult for this group of children, as a result of several factors, e.g. decreased sense of thirst, inability to let others know they are thirsty, poor swallowing skills associated with risk of aspiration on thin fluids. There may also be additional fluid losses through excessive drooling, secondary to poor lip seal or an inability to manage saliva secretions or over active salivary gland. Nevertheless, some of these children may, in reality, be able to remain well on a lower fluid intake than the estimated requirements. Keeping an eye on the number of wet nappies in a day, as well as the consistency of stool output could help to ascertain if additional fluids will be required.

Table 4.2 Fluid requirements based on body weight for children on liquid diet only[29]

Body weight range (kg)	Fluid requirements
2–8	150 ml/kg/d
6–10	120 ml/kg/d
11–20	1000 ml + 50 ml/kg for next 10 kg
20 kg and above	1500 ml + 25 ml/kg thereafter, up to 2500 ml/d

Table 4.3 Dietary Reference Values (DRV) for fluid for children consuming a mixed diet[29]

Age	Fluid requirements (ml/kg/d)
0–6 months	150
7–12 months	120
1–3 years	90
4–6 years	80
7–10 years	60
11–14 years	50
15–18 years	40

Role of essential fatty acids

Essential fatty acids (EFA), the omega-6 (alpha-linolenic acid) and the omega-3 (linoleic acid) fatty acids, cannot be synthesized within the body and must be ingested from dietary sources in order to meet the requirements of individuals. Although the omega-6 (*n-6*) fatty acids can be found in abundance in most diets, the omega-3 (*n-3*) family is less common but is found in selected nuts and predominantly fish.

In the last decade, much attention has centred on the *n-3* long-chain polyunsaturated fatty acid, docosahexaenoic acid (DHA), and their role in the central nervous system. It is recognized that DHA is the main ingredient required for fetal brain development *in utero* and has long-term benefits for neurodevelopment in children. The knowledge surrounding the role of DHA in brain development has largely been derived from studies involving preterm and term infants, who may not have been neurologically compromised. Potential benefits for neurosystem disorders have been suggested by several studies showing positive effects of *n-3* fatty acids supplementation in children with learning difficulties, dyslexia, dyspraxia.[30] Studies in Alzheimer's disease identified a possible protective role for DHA in neurodegenerative disorders and brain ischaemia, possibly through promoting neuronal survival and nerve growth.[31] *n-3* fatty acids are central components of the brain and take part in brain membrane remodelling and synthesis, with DHA in particular, essential for myelin formation.[31] Extrapolating the hypothesis to children with neurological impairment is plausible, given that different epidemiological studies have pointed towards diets enriched in *n-3* fatty acids having neuroprotective effects.[31]

With the high incidence of feeding problems, children with neurological impairment represent a group who may be at risk of EFA deficiency. Hals et al investigated the dietary intakes and serum phospholipids concentrations of EFA in a group of children with severe neurological impairment.[32] Dietary intakes were found to be suboptimal (0.37% of energy intake for *n-3* fatty acids), which corresponded with low serum concentrations; however, the serum levels improved to normal levels after supplementation with 5 g fish oils equivalent to 0.44 g eicosapentaenoic acid (EPA) and 0.52g DHA.[32] According to the European Union reference intake recommendations (1993) 2% of dietary energy should be derived from *n-6* fatty acids and 0.5% from *n-3* fatty acids for children above 4 years of age (equivalent to 4 g of *n-6* fatty acids and 1 g of *n-3* fatty acids in relation to body weight, energy or protein intakes). However, the appropriateness of the recommended dietary allowances that are based on the percentage of total dietary energy intake, for children with neurological impairment, is debateable, taking into consideration their risk of a lower total dietary energy intake compared with other children. Although Hals et al proposed that the serum levels should be monitored for the adequacy of EFA intake, it is not practically realistic to do so.[32] Thus, until further evidence and recommendations emerge, the percentage of dietary energy from EFA or the calculation of absolute intakes of EFA must be used.

Common nutrient deficiencies

As the energy requirement of children with neurological impairment is often reduced, they can possibly be at risk of micronutrient deficiencies. Studies have reported deficient intakes of iron, copper, zinc, selenium, folate, niacin, vitamin C, D and E.[17,33,34] Biochemical analyses in the studies by Hals et al[33] and Hillesund et al[34] showed corresponding low serum levels of ferritin, selenium, zinc, folate, vitamin E and D. However, there were no signs of protein inadequacy in the diets of the children with varying degrees of neurodisability.[33,34]

As highlighted in Chapter 3, children with neurodevelopmental disability commonly have feeding difficulties such as oral motor difficulties, oropharyngeal difficulties and swallowing problems which will impact their ability to eat and drink. The Oxford Feeding Study emphasized the prevalence of feeding problems:

- 89% needed help with feeding;
- 56% choked with food;
- 28% reported feeding took longer than 3 hours per day.[35]

In addition, 64% of the children in the Oxford Feeding Study had never had any feeding or nutrition assessment. It is obvious that any feeding difficulties are likely to have an impact on the dietary intake and hence nutritional status. The dietitian involved in the care of such children needs to remember the importance of determining the food actually eaten versus reportedly offered.

Choice of foods in the diet will clearly have an effect on nutrient intake. The Oxford Feeding Study showed that milk and milk-based drinks provided the highest proportion of energy for most of the children with severe disabilities; thus the micronutrient profile was biased towards those abundant in dairy products, like protein, calcium and phosphorus. It was deficient in nutrients found in foods parents reportedly excluded from the diet because of feeding problems, such as meat (rich sources of iron and zinc), fruits and vegetables (sources of folate, vitamin A and C).[17]

The prolonged use of anticonvulsant therapy in children with neurological impairment has been associated with alterations in vitamin D and calcium metabolism.[25,27] However, other factors, such as limited ambulation and reduced sun exposure may contribute to the prevalence of osteopenia in these children.[25] Therefore, their calcium and vitamin D intakes should be carefully monitored to ensure healthy bone development.

Given the difficulties with ensuring a well-balanced diet for these children, it is not surprising that orally fed children can develop micronutrient deficiencies. However, the possibility of developing micronutrient deficiencies when being fed on enteral formulae is also not unconceivable. Stathopolou and Thomas found that the abnormal serum levels of micronutrients were not confined to those who were clinically malnourished, but also in five children who had previously been started on 'nutritionally complete' enteral feeds via gastrostomy.[36] As enteral formulae are formulated to provide adequate amounts of micronutrients when the volume consumed meet their age-related dietary reference intake for energy,[25] children who are fed less volume because of lower energy requirements than the average population can become deficient in certain micronutrients.

In contrast however, Johnson et al found, in a observational study of children aged 1–6 years who were receiving supplemental nutrition support, no significant micronutrient deficiencies on blood analysis.[37] Instead, 83% and 92% had high vitamin B_{12} and copper intake above 150% of the RNI respectively and it was despite a median energy intake of 75% EAR. The study demonstrated that not only is it possible for micronutrient status to be maintained, it is also possible for a child on supplemental enteral feeds to develop micronutrient excesses. Attention is often focused on avoiding nutritional deficiencies but the potential of micronutrient toxicity should also be considered.

Dietary approaches to optimizing nutrition

The nutrition of many children with neurological impairment is often neglected yet they need a diet that is as nutritious as that of their peers without neurological impairment. For this reason, the meals of children who have functional oropharyngeal skills that allow them to consume a normal diet should be made up of a variety of foods from the four major food groups – bread, other cereals and potatoes; fruits and vegetables; meat, fish and alternatives; milk and dairy foods. In the UK, the 'Eat Well Plate' (www.eatwell.gov.uk/healthydiet/eatwellplate/) guides the recommended balance of foods for a well balanced diet, whereas the USA uses the pyramid model (http://myPyramid.gov).

Table 4.4 provides examples of foods and the major nutrients found in each group. Foods containing additional fat and sugar may not be essential; nonetheless such foods can add variety and improve the palatability of foods. These foods are frequently discouraged for the healthy population. Ironically, there may be a role for these foods in this group of children who may often struggle to consume a diet adequate in calories. The physical barriers, such as fatigue and lethargy during meals, or coughing and choking on food may shorten mealtimes, thus preventing these children from receiving the nutrition they need. The presence of spillage, and/or frequent large vomits would also have an impact on their actual food intake. Feeding has been described by Sullivan et al as being stressful and unenjoyable for parents and carers and feeding times prolonged.[35] To try to increase portion sizes or the frequency of feeding may prove to be a challenging task for those who encounter feeding problems. Therefore, utilizing high energy foods, such as full fat dairy products, as discussed briefly in Chapter 3, is a practical solution.

Table 4.4 Major food groups in a balanced diet

Food group	Bread, other cereals and potatoes	Fruits and vegetables	Meat, fish and alternatives	Milk and dairy foods
Examples	bread, rolls, chapatti, breakfast cereals, oats, pasta, rice, noodles, potatoes, yam, plantain, cornmeal, millet	all fresh, frozen and tinned fruits and vegetables, 100% fruit juices, dried fruits	meat (beef, lamb, pork, bacon), poultry (chicken, turkey), fresh or frozen or canned fish, meat products e.g. sausages and burgers, fish products e.g. fish fingers and fish cakes, eggs, beans and lentils including baked beans and chickpeas, nuts, textured vegetable protein, soy products e.g. tofu, soy mince	milk, cheese, yogurt, fromage frais
Good sources of:	carbohydrate, B vitamins and some iron (especially whole-grains and whole-meal versions)	vitamin C, beta-carotene (vitamin A), folate, some iron and calcium (in dark green vegetables), fibre, some carbohydrate	protein, iron, zinc, B vitamins	calcium, protein, vitamins B_{12}, A and D

Table 4.5 Overview of foods available to enhance energy, protein, vitamins A, D, E, folate, iron, zinc, selenium and fibre in the diet

Food	Calories	Protein	Vit A	Vit D	Vit E	Folate	Iron	Zinc	Selenium	Fibre
Red meat/poultry	✓	✓					✓	✓	✓	
Fish	✓	✓		✓ (oily fish)[a]					✓	
Egg	✓	✓		✓			✓		✓	
Cheese	✓	✓	✓	✓				✓	✓	
Cream cheese	✓	✓	✓							
Tofu		✓					✓	✓		
Beans		✓							✓	✓
Mushrooms		✓							✓	
Nuts	✓	✓			✓ (hazel-nuts)	✓ (pea-nuts)		✓	✓ (Brazil nuts)	✓
Liver			✓				✓		✓	
Margarine/butter	✓		✓	✓						
Double cream	✓		✓							
Orange-fleshed veg			✓							✓
Avocado	✓		✓		✓	✓	✓			
Yeast/meat extract						✓	✓	✓		
Wheat germ/bran						✓	✓	✓		✓
Seeds	✓						✓	✓		✓
Pine nuts	✓	✓					✓	✓		
Wholemeal bread							✓		✓	✓
Houmous							✓		✓	
Miso (Japanese)									✓	

a. Oily fish includes kippers, tinned salmon, herring, pilchards, sardines and mackerel.

Before considering the use of proprietary dietary supplements, fortifying foods at home should be encouraged for the group of children who are able to be fed orally. Table 4.5 (page 77) gives an overview of the foods that can be used to enhance the energy, protein and the known 'at risk' micronutrients, as well as fibre.

As discussed in Chapter 3, some children may require a texture modification determined by their oropharyngeal skills, thus limiting their ability to cope with the variety of foods necessary to achieve an optimal nutritional balance. They may only be able to deal with, for example, a smooth puréed consistency of a specific viscosity. Preparing suitable foods can become time consuming and demanding for the parents or carers, and may result in meals consisting of a single ingredient, such as mashed potatoes or porridge oats. Moreover, the nutrient density of puréed meals is frequently diluted down with the addition of liquids in the process to obtain the correct texture. As a consequence children can gradually become malnourished on a poorly planned puréed diet. This can also happen if children are solely (or even partially, but regularly) fed on commercially available puréed foods sold for the purpose of weaning of infants

Table 4.6 Examples of using common foods to optimize energy and protein density

Typical Meal Plan[a]		Modifications	Energy and protein added
Breakfast	1 small bowl (110 g) oatmeal porridge[b] with milk	+ 30 ml double cream + 30 g ground almonds	104 kcal 180 kcal, 7.0 g protein
Lunch	1 medium bowl (200 g) Tomato soup	+ 30 ml double cream + 100 g baked beans, mashed	104 kcal 98 kcal, 7.2 g protein
Mid-afternoon	Milk (240 ml)	+ 1 small avocado to blend	190 kcal, 1.9 g protein
Dinner	2 scoops (120 g) mash potatoes with butter and milk	+ 30 ml double cream + 1/2 hard-boiled egg, mashed + 30 g grated cheese	104 kcal 44 kcal, 3.8 g protein 125 kcal, 7.6 g protein
Nutrients	**Typical meal plan provides**	**Modifications add**	**Final meal plan provides**
Energy (kcal)	511	949	1460
Protein (g)	17.1	27.5	44.6

a. Average portion size for a young child. Portion sizes may vary.
b. Choose fortified cereals where available, e.g. ReadyBrek, Oatibix, Weetabix.

onto solid foods. These products are not nutritionally complete and either completely lack many of the micronutrients essential for health or will not provide appropriate intakes. As an example, one of the authors of this chapter (BL) was involved with a child with neurological impairment who had a significant feeding problem and had been fed exclusively for several years on 10–12 jars daily of a sweet pudding designed for weaning infants. Although his weight was satisfactory, the micronutrient content of his diet was severely compromised. When first reviewed in clinic he was suffering from a range of symptoms of frank clinical deficiencies of vitamins and minerals, notably vitamin C (scurvy), iron (anaemia) and vitamin A (xeropthalmia) among others.

Thus, ways to incorporate nutrient-dense foods over and above the mere mention of the foods available, should be discussed with parents or carers (See Appendix 4). Tables 4.6 and 4.7 illustrate a few examples of how common foods can be used to optimize the energy/nutrient density. However, it may not always be possible to fortify the diet with

Table 4.7 Examples of using common foods to optimize iron and zinc density

Typical Meal Plan[a]		Modifications	Energy and protein added
Breakfast	1 small bowl (100 g) oatmeal porridge[b] with milk	Choose fortified cereals	Up to 12.5 mg iron, 1.7 mg zinc[c]
Lunch	1 medium bowl (200 g) Tomato soup	+ 30 g minced meat (blend as required)	0.7 mg iron, 1.5 mg zinc
Mid-afternoon	Milk (240 ml)	+ 1 tablespoon wheatgerm	0.9 mg iron, 1.7 mg zinc
Dinner	2 scoops (120 g) mash potatoes with butter and milk	+ 2 tablespoons houmous	1.1 mg iron, 0.8 mg zinc
		+ gravy, with 2 teaspoons meat extract added	0.8 mg iron, 0.2 mg zinc
			3.8 mg iron, 4.2 mg zinc
Nutrients	**Typical meal plan provides**	**Modifications will add**	**Final meal plan provides**
Iron (mg)	1.8	3.8	5.6 (92% RNI)[d]
Zinc (mg)	2.7	4.2	6.9 (106% RNI)[d]

a. Average portion size for a young child. Portion sizes may vary.
b. Choose fortified cereals where available, e.g. ReadyBrek, Oatibix, Weetabix.
c. Values not added into final meal plan.
d. Reference nutrient intakes for 4–6-year-old child.

common foods. It can be particularly difficult to introduce new tastes to children with neurological dysfunction, as they may have low sensory tolerance. Thus, even a slight tweak of the diet can upset them and lead to problems of rejection. Compared with a child with no sensory defensiveness, more time and effort will be needed for them to learn to accept anything new. If fortified or enriched products are available, most commonly breakfast cereals, substituting non-fortified foods with them should be encouraged. Otherwise, if all else fails with food fortification, proprietary energy supplements (See Appendix 5), e.g. Super Soluble Duocal (SHS) or Super Soluble Maxijul (SHS), would then be useful. Such products can be easily incorporated into foods and drinks, without significantly altering their tastes or consistencies. However, the tendency to use these products due to the ease and increased acceptability will mean that they can potentially be used excessively, even at the expense of nutritional foods. Although there are no definite guidelines for their safe usage, in our clinical experience, 40–50 g per day of Duocal or Maxijul, given distributed over several feeds, has been tolerated. Nevertheless, tolerance will differ between individuals, so the dose should be adjusted accordingly by a dietitian or clinician. The option of administering vitamin and/or mineral supplements (See Appendix 5) may also become necessary for some children.

Constipation can be an issue for children with neurological impairment and is generally because of reduced gut motility.[38] It can also be related to poor fluid and dietary fibre intake. Incorporating sources of fibre into a child's diet such as fruits, vegetables, pulses, ground nuts and cereals, in addition to trying to improve fluid intake, can be very helpful in some cases.

Enteral feeding

The process of deciding to feed a child with neurological impairment using a tube and the associated practicalities of this are described in Chapter 5 of this book.

With regard to the choice of a particular formula for an individual, there are many options available here in the United Kingdom (Appendix 5, Tables 1, 2, 5, 6 and 7). They are prescribable based on age and weight, and their nutritional content formulated accordingly. It is important that the child's nutritional requirements be adequately met, not just for energy and macronutrients but also for micronutrients. As discussed previously in this chapter, estimating these can be difficult, particularly for energy, which may be much reduced, compared with normal age requirements. Hence, a low energy feed may be indicated or a small volume of an energy dense feed if this is better tolerated. Micronutrient intakes should be matched to age DRVs.[19] To ensure these are achieved, it may be preferable to use an adult feed even for young children or add in a supplement such as Paediatric Seravit (Appendix 5, Table 8). If the child has a history of constipation, a feed containing fibre is preferable. The majority of children with neurological impairment will tolerate a whole protein (polymeric) feed, but if there are problems with feed tolerance or food allergy then a semi-elemental or elemental formula may be indicated (Appendix 5, Tables 6 and 7). Regular review of nutritional intake is vital to ensure appropriate growth is taking place and the tube fed child is meeting their requirements for micronutrients. For further information on enteral feeding for children with neurological impairments see for example Johnson[39] and Almond et al.[26]

In the UK using foods that have been blended down to feed children who have a gastrostomy is not routinely practised or recommended by dietitians. However, in other parts of the world, children with a gastrostomy are fed normal, everyday foods that have been modified to a liquid or semi-solid consistency, or a combination of foods mixed with enteral feeds might be given. A search on the internet reveals a couple of websites which offer advice on giving food via a gastrostomy (for example: www.kidswithtubes.org and www.mealtimenotions.com). Both emphasize that the involvement of a trained dietitian is of utmost importance. This is to help ensure that nutritional adequacy is maintained and individual dietary requirements met if foods as opposed to formulas are given.

There are valid justifications and reasons for the use of either foods or formulas, or a combination, to nourish a tube fed individual. This section will consider the advantages and disadvantages of both of these practices. It is worth pointing out that if blended foods are used they are best given via a gastrostomy. This is because they may more easily clog a nasogastric tube which is generally narrower and more prone to blocking.

Advantages of using enteral formulas

- The enteral feeds available for tube feeding, both in the UK (on prescription) and worldwide have been formulated against strict nutritional standards and regulations (for example, the European Union Commission Directive N° 1999/21/EC of 25 March 1999 on Dietary Foods for Special Medical Purposes (amended by Directive 2006/141/EC)).
- Their nutritional content is known and the information made available.
- Many have been designed to meet the specific dietary requirements of children.
- Provided they are prescribed appropriately and their use monitored (preferably by a trained dietitian) they can be relied upon to meet nutritional requirements adequately and safely in terms of intakes of macro- and micronutrients.
- Most of the formulas currently available have been in regular use in the UK for a number of years. Thus, there is a history of their use in terms of efficacy (for example, in the promotion of growth) and tolerance, both in the short and long term.
- Prescribable enteral formulas designed to be nutritionally complete can be used as a sole source of nutrition.
- Enteral feeds have been designed with a viscosity such that they generally go down tubes easily.
- Enteral feeds are available with different energy contents per ml of feed, e.g. 1 kcal/ml, 1.5 kcal/ml and this flexibility can be useful. For example, if a child cannot tolerate 750 ml of a 1 kcal/ml feed they may be more comfortable on 500 ml of a 1.5 kcal/ml feed, yet will still have the same energy intake.

- Ready to feed preparations are sterile, easy to use and in the majority of cases will not require any modification (e.g. addition of extra ingredients) for the recipient.
- Feeds that are only available in a powder form will require time spent in preparation compared with ready to use presentations, yet will have all the nutritional advantages of liquid feeds.
- Provided they are stored correctly before and after opening and/or preparation, formulas are safe microbiologically and their nutritional content can be relied upon (unless the manufacturer has identified a quality control problem and subsequently is obliged to withdraw the product!).

Disadvantages of enteral formulas

- The foods we eat contain many components and micronutrients known to be essential to good health and development. Equally there are substances in foods that are either unknown or have as yet no recognized purpose in the body.
- Despite advances in the formulation of enteral feeds, particularly over the past 10 years, formulas do not include all the different and varied components that foods are naturally composed of.
- Some substances found naturally in foods considered important to the correct functioning of the body and for the long-term prevention of disease (such as antioxidants and bioflavonoids) cannot, at present, be included in manufactured feeds. This is for a variety of reasons, such as European Union legislation prohibiting their use, the non-stability of the substance in a feed or because there is a lack of evidence to support safe use or the appropriate level to add to a formula.
- This then means that the enteral feeds currently available, although they provide the micronutrients known to be essential to correct functioning of the body and in amounts considered appropriate, cannot be relied upon to provide absolutely everything that a normal varied diet can. Hence, inadvertently, individuals fed enteral formulas long term, particularly as a sole source of nutrition, could potentially miss out on certain components naturally occurring in food that may in some way be essential to their health and well-being. But whether this is of significance to a greater or lesser degree is as yet unknown.
- Gut flora – those individuals fed solely on sterile ready to feed preparations will, unlike those consuming a normal diet, not be taking in bacteria which may affect the normal functioning of the gut. However, there are enteral feeds that contain fibre that tend to be used in children with neurological impairment to prevent constipation. These often have a prebiotic component (e.g. fructo-oligosaccharides) which may contribute to the maintenance and proliferation of a health gut flora. Children could be given probiotic preparations, such as live yogurt or capsules of bacteria to ensure an intake of probiotic if this was considered desirable.
- Enteral feeds are expensive. In the UK 'free' prescriptions are available for children yet there is obviously a price to be paid by the National Health Service. In countries where medical care is not provided by the state then people will be required to pay for feeds themselves.

Advantages of using foods

- Using foods prepared and usually eaten within the home may be considered as more 'natural' than opening a bottle of a ready prepared formula. Hence, caregivers may perceive the blending down of food that will also be consumed by others in the family as a more acceptable and preferred way of providing nourishment to their child. The desire to feed and nurture a child can not be underestimated, in addition to the concept of the child then being able to share foods that others are eating, for example at family mealtimes. Many parents, in the experience of the author BL, do miss preparing food for the child that was once fed orally but who now is reliant on formula given via a gastrostomy.
- Caregivers may feel they have more control over what their child has to eat when preparing their own foods rather than giving them the same formula feeds all the time. The fact that the child will not taste the food as it will go straight into the stomach via the gastrostomy is not of importance to them.
- Provided care is taken with the balance of foods used and nutritional adequacy calculated a blended food diet can potentially meet dietary requirements. Ideally, a dietitian should be involved to analyse recipes and ensure dietary requirements are met. This should be carried out on a regular basis.
- Foods can be combined with enteral formulas and/or to ensure optimal nutritional intake.

Disadvantages of using foods

- Preparing blended foods can be time consuming and messy.
- Time is also needed to ensure foods are prepared and stored hygienically to prevent contamination and illness.
- Liquidized food needs 'thinning' with additional fluid to get down the gastrostomy tube. Even if a nutritious fluid such as milk is used this may have the effect of dilute the nutrient content of the meal, or altering the balance of nutrients present.
- Large volumes of blended foods may be required to meet nutritional requirements because of the food components not being viscous enough to pass down the tube easily without the addition of lots of extra fluid. This may then be uncomfortable for the child who may not be able to accommodate all the food needed to ensure they meet their nutritional requirements.
- Cooking and the process of the preparation of meals can cause losses of nutrients from foods although in contrast it enhances some.
- Reliance on milk-based foods for a blended diet means that without careful consideration dietary inadequacy or imbalance can result.
- More dietetic time is required to assess dietary intake and adequacy.
- Blockages are more likely with the use of blended and liquidized foods, for example, because of meat fibres, fibre from vegetables and starch grains from foods such as potatoes.

- The manufacturers of gastrostomy tubes have not generally designed them to be used to give food rather than enteral formulas. A tube that is frequently blocked will eventually need replacing with associated cost implications.
- Potentially, the use of blended foods that are obviously not as sterile as enteral feeds may increase the risk of bacteria infecting the gastrostomy site and tract.

It is the personal practice of both authors of this chapter to use the specially formulated enteral feeds that are available for children fed via a gastrostomy (or nasogastric tube), and recommend and advocate their use to health professionals and parents accordingly. However, children fed solely by a tube should, if it is safe to do, be given opportunity to have some food by mouth to allow them to experience taste.

References

1. Reilly JJ, Hassan TM, Braekken A, Jolly J, Day RE. Growth retardation and undernutrition in children with spastic cerebral palsy. *J Hum Nutr and Diet* 1996; **9**: 429–35.
2. Fung EB, Samson-Fang L, Stallings VA et al. Feeding dysfunction is associated with poor growth and health status in children with cerebral palsy. *J Am Diet Assoc* 2002; **102**: 3–73.
3. Troughton KE, Hill AE. Relation between objectively measured feeding competence and nutrition in children with cerebral palsy. *Dev Med Child Neurol* 2001; **43**: 187–90.
4. USDA/FNS – FNS-253. *Feeding Infants: A Guide for Use in the Child Care Food Program.* USDA/FNS, December 1983. Available at: www.fcs.uga.edu/pubs/PDF/FDNS-NE-1405.pdf
5. Butte NF, Hopkinson JM, Wong WW, Smith EO, Ellis KJ. Body composition during the first 2 years of life: an updated reference. *Pediatr Res* 2000; **47**: 578–85.
6. Sullivan PB, Rosenbloom L. *Feeding the Disabled Child.* London: MacKeith Press, 1996.
7. Craig GM, Scambler G, Spitz L. Why parents of children with neurodevelopmental disabilities requiring gastrostomy feeding need more support. *Dev Med Child Neurol* 2003; **45**: 183–8.
8. Chailey Heritage Clinical Services. *Eating and Drinking Skills for Children with Motor Disorders.* Lewes: Chailey Heritage Clinical Services, 1998.
9. Kostraba JN, Dorman JS, LaPorte RE et al. Early infant diet and risk of IDDM in blacks and whites. A matched case-control study. *Diabetes Care* 1992; **15**: 626–31.
10. Adams RA, Gordon C, Spangler AA. Maternal stress in caring for children with feeding disabilities: implications for health care providers. *J Am Diet Assoc* 1999; **99**: 8–6.
11. Sullivan PB, Lambert B, Rose M, Ford-Adams M, Griffiths P, Johnson A. An epidemiological study of feeding and nutritional problems in children with neurological impairment. *J Pediatr Gastroenterol Nutr* 1998; **26**: 587–A244.
12. Sullivan PB, Rosenbloom L. An overview of the feeding difficulties experienced by disabled children. In: Sullivan PB, Rosenbloom L, editors. *Feeding the Disabled Child.* London: MacKeith Press, 1996. pp. 1–10.
13. Tawfik R, Dickson A, Clarke M, Thomas AG. Caregivers' perceptions following gastrostomy in severely disabled children with feeding problems. *Dev Med Child Neurol* 1997; **39**: 746–51.
14. Gisel EG, Patrick J. Identification of children with cerebral palsy unable to maintain a normal nutritional state. *Lancet* 1988; **1**: 283–6.
15. Thomas B. Dietary assessment. In: Thomas B, Bishop J, editors. *Manual of Dietetic Practice,* 4th edn. Ofxofrd: Blackwell Publishing, 2007.
16. Stallings V, Babette A, Zemel S et al. Energy expenditure of children and adolescents with severe disabilities: a cerebral palsy model. *Am J Clin Nutr* 1996; **64**: 627–34.
17. Sullivan PB, Juszczak E, Lambert BR, Rose M, Ford-Adams ME, Johnson A. Impact of feeding problems on nutritional intake and growth: Oxford feeding study II. *Dev Med Child Neurol* 2002; **44**: 461–7.

18. Stewart, L, McKaig N, Dunlop C, Daly H, Almond S. *Professional Concensus Statement. Dietetic Assessment and Monitoring of Children with Special Needs with Faltering Growth*. Birmingham: British Dietetic Association Specialist Paediatric Group, 2002.
19. Department of Health. *Report on Health and Social Subjects No. 41. Dietary Reference Values for Food Energy and Nutrients fo the United Kingdom*. London: The Stationery Office. 1991.
20. Bandini LG, Schoeller DA, Fukagawa NK, Wykes LJ, Dietz WH. Body composition and energy expenditure in adolescents with cerebral palsy or myelodysplasia. *Pediatric Research* 1991; **29**: 70–77.
21. Bandini LG, Puelzl-Quinn H, Morelli JA, Fukagawa NK. Estimation of energy requirements in persons with severe central nervous system impairment. *J Pediatr* 1995; **126**: 828–32.
22. Sullivan PB, Alder N, Bachlet AM et al. Gastrostomy feeding in cerebral palsy: too much of a good thing? *Dev Med Child Neurol* 2006; **48**: 877–82.
23. Krick J, Murphy PE, Markham JFB, Shapiro BK. A proposed formula for calculating energy needs of children with cerebral palsy. *Dev Med Child Neurol* 1992; **34**: 481–7.
24. Culley WJ, Middleton TO. Caloric requirements of mentally retarded children with and without motor dysfunction. J Pediatr 1969; **75**: 380–4.
25. Marchand V, Motil KJ and the NASPGHAN Committee on Nutrition. Nutrition support for neurologically impaired children: a clinical report of the North American society for pediatric gastroenterology, hepatology and nutrition. *J Pediatr Gastroenterol Nutr* 2006; **43**: 123–135.
26. Almond, S, Allot L, Hall K. Feeding Children with neurodisabilities. In: Shaw V, Lawson M, editors. *Clinical Paediatric Dietetics*. Oxford: Blackwell Publishing, 2007.
27. Bandini, L, Ekvall SW, Stallings, S. Cerebral palsy. In: Shaw V, Lawson M, editors. *Pediatric Nutrition in Chronic Diseases and Developmental Disorders*. Oxford: Oxford University Press, 2005.
28. Food and Nutritional Board, Institute of Medicine, National Academies. *Dietary Reference Intakes (DRIs): Recommended Intakes for Individuals*. National Academy of Science, 2004. http://fnic.nal.usda.gov/nal_display/index.php?info_center=4&tax_level=3&tax_subject=256&topic_id=1342&level3_id=5140&level4_id=0&level5_id=0&placement_default=0
29. Shaw V, Lawson M. Nutritional assessment, dietary requirements, feed supplementation. In Shaw V, Lawson M, editors. *Clinical Paediatric Dietetics*. Oxford: Blackwell Publishing, 2007. pp. 566–87.
30. Genuis SJ, Schwalfenberg GK. Time for an oil check: the role of essential omega-3 fatty acids in maternal and pediatric health. *J Perinatol* 2006; **26**: 359–65.
31. Mazza, M, Pomponi M, Janiri L, Bria P, Mazza S. Omega-3 fatty acids and antioxidants in neurological and psychiatric diseases: an overview. *Prog Neuropyschopharmacol Biol Pyschiatry* 2000; **31**: 12–26.
32. Hals J, Bjerve KS, Nilsen H, Svalastog AG, Ek J. Essential fatty acids in the nutrition of severely neurologically disabled children. *Br J Nutr* 2000; **83**: 219–25.
33. Hals J, Ek J, Svalastog AG, Nilsen, H. Studies on nutrition in severely neurologically disabled children in an institution. *Acta Paediatr* 1996; **85**: 1469–75.
34. Hillesund E, Skranes J, Trygg KU, Bohmer T. Micronutrient status in children with cerebral palsy. *Acta Paediatr* 2007; **96**: 1195–8.
35. Sullivan PB, Lambert B, Rose M, Ford-Adams M. Johnson A, Griffiths P. Prevalence and severity of feeding and nutritional problems in children with neurological impairment: Oxford feeding study. *Dev Med Child Neurol* 2000; **42**: 674–80.
36. Stathopolou E, Thomas AG. Nutrition in disabled children. *Acta Paediatr* 1997; **86**: 670.
37. Johnson TE, Janes SJ, MacDonald A, Elia M, Booth IW. An observational study to evaluate micronutrient status during enteral feeding. *Arch Dis Child* 2002; **86**: 411–15.
38. Sullivan PB. Gastrointestinal disorders in children with neurodevelopment disabilities. *Dev Disabil Res Rev* 2008; **14**: 128–36.
39. Johnson T. Enteral nutrition. In: Shaw V, Lawson M, editors. *Clinical Paediatric Dietetics*. Oxford: Blackwell Publishing, 2007.

Chapter 5

The Multidisciplinary Team and the Practicalities of Nursing Care

Angharad Vernon-Roberts

Introduction

The nutritional management of children with neurological impairment is a complex mosaic of physical, psychological, social, emotional and environmental factors. The feeding process begins when a child anticipates and prepares to receive food or liquid and ends with digestion and elimination.[1] Feeding disorders develop when this progression is disrupted, and the efficacy of any therapeutic intervention relies fundamentally on understanding the diverse elements of the process.

There are many areas that need to be addressed when planning nutritional intervention for a child with neurological impairment. This chapter is concerned specifically with the nurse's role in the preparation, safety and comfort of the child and family and the following areas are considered:

- multidisciplinary team coordination
- behavioural issues
- enteral nutrition: the practicalities
- support
- training
- health promotion
- dental health
- intervention planning

Multidisciplinary team coordination

Multidisciplinary team work is essential for the assessment of a child's needs and the prescription, administration and monitoring of clinical treatment.[2] Feeding is a complex physiological process and when it goes awry a unified treatment strategy is required. This should involve professionals from various disciplines who can between them provide all the necessary skills and knowledge to manage feeding difficulties. Specific multidisciplinary feeding teams and clinics have been established in many centres and ideally should incorporate input from the following professionals:

- paediatric gastroenterologist;
- paediatric surgeon;
- community paediatrician;
- family doctor;
- paediatric radiologist;
- clinical nurse specialist;
- dietitian;
- speech and language therapist;
- physiotherapist;
- occupational therapist;
- psychologist;
- play therapist;
- social workers;
- community nurse;
- health visitor;
- school.

It is traditionally the consultant's responsibility to coordinate and oversee the activities of the multidisciplinary team.[2] The nurse also plays an important role in implementing many of the strategies and solutions that may have been put in place. The multidisciplinary team will work more effectively and provide a better service to the families if there is one main person who coordinates information between professionals. The child's best interests are served if there is close cooperation and a flexible cross-disciplinary approach between all team members, especially when so many specialities are intertwined.[3] The aim of multidisciplinary teamwork should be to provide effective treatment and open, balanced communication between all the necessary hospital and community based resources. The team should be able to take on responsibility for the following aspects of support:[2]

- provide an effective advisory service at district/hospital level;
- identify those patients requiring nutritional support;
- implement and evaluate nutritional support;
- provide a specialist service for placement of feeding tubes;
- develop policies that are, as far as possible, evidenced-based, in accordance with nutritional and local guidelines;

- develop programmes for patient education in conjunction with the wards and the family or carers;
- provide teaching, education and support for family, school and respite care;
- provide in-service continuing education updates on clinical nutrition to staff.

Parents or primary carers should also be considered valuable members of the multidisciplinary team. They play a vital role in the delivery and success of any treatment plan and should be invited to participate in all meetings concerning their child.[3] Providing information and participating in discussions will promote understanding of the reasons for commencing nutritional support, and helps facilitate informed participation in decision-making. This will, in turn, maximize the efficiency and effectiveness of any feeding plan implemented.

Behavioural issues

The prevalence of emotional disorders and behavioural problems is significantly higher in children with neurological impairments and these frequently manifest as feeding difficulties.[1] Behaviour mismanagement is the primary factor associated with more than 21% of all feeding problems in disabled children referred to tertiary clinics.[1] Behavioural problems that are experienced during feeding can be associated with both child and adult orientated factors, such as anxiety, control, anticipation and expectation.[4]

When a child has problems with eating and drinking, mealtimes can become difficult for all those involved, and may be unrewarding and not enjoyable for the carer and child. The carer is faced with many conflicting demands that occur alongside ensuring adequate nutrition and a balanced intake for growth and health. Accounts of feeding given by parents and carers are often ambivalent and contradictory using militaristic metaphors (war, battle, torture), although also saying feeding time is 'special' for bonding, closeness and the child's pleasure and enjoyment.[5]

Barriers to feeding

There are a number of behavioural factors that may be detrimental to the feeding process and these must be identified before any intervention takes place. The issues may be child or carer based and should be addressed, as outlined below:

- disability;
- medical factors;
- agitation;
- lethargy;
- aversion to feeding;
- communication problems;
- feeding interactions;
- parents/carers.

Disability

When caring for children with neurological impairments and feeding difficulties, it is crucial to look beyond their disability and make sure that their 'special needs' do not overshadow their 'ordinary needs', which should not be overlooked. The multidisciplinary team must take a positive outlook and think about what each child *can* do rather than that which they cannot.[3] A good relationship between the multidisciplinary team and the parents and carers is essential. Parents are the experts at caring for their child and can tell you how (and how not) to manage their child, including behavioural boundaries, likes and dislikes.[3] It is important to make certain that all carers communicate with the children directly and ask how they would like to be moved, positioned and helped with eating and drinking. The physiotherapist or occupational therapist can provide practical help and advice to ensure that they are supported and comfortable at all times.[3]

Medical factors

Feeding is a multisystem skill that requires structural integrity, neuromuscular control and coordination, and sensory perception.[1] The child must also have adequate gastrointestinal function, cardiorespiratory support and integration from the autonomic nervous system.[1] When feeding problems occur it is important to consider that they may be as a result of respiratory distress, a dysfunctional swallow, pain from gastro-oesophageal reflux (GOR) or oral lesions due to dental problems.

Agitation

It is very easy to misinterpret a child's symptoms of agitation such as crying, hyperextension and refusal to sit in their chair. These could be a result of a medical problem such as pain from GOR, discomfort from constipation or from a behavioural issue such as lack of hunger, positioning problems or that they do not want the meal being offered.[1] Central nervous system abnormalities may also result in a child's inability to filter sensory input and/or modulate their responses to situations.

Lethargy

For oral feeding to result in adequate nutrition, the child must be an active participant by being awake, calm and cooperative. Sleepiness and lethargy can interfere greatly with feeding and intake; this may have a specific medical cause, and the effect of medications should also be considered.

The length of mealtimes should be controlled so that the child does not become excessively tired. This is also important for the carer so that the child's disabilities that prolong feeding do not cause them to become bored and uninterested, thus giving negative messages to the child.

Aversion to feeding

Adults know the importance of adequate nutrition, but children have different motivating factors such as pleasure from taste and sensation, social interaction and relief of hunger. If these motivators are impaired and if oral feeding is difficult for the child, then maladaptive feeding behaviours such as food refusal may be observed.[1] Eating may not be a pleasurable experience and aversion becomes learned from experience. The sights, sounds, textures and smells of feeding may be associated with pain, discomfort from GOR, choking, aspiration and difficulty in satisfying hunger.

Communication problems

Children with severe language and communication difficulties can be at risk of undernutrition and dehydration as they may not be able to indicate when they are hungry and thirsty. When caring for a child who does not find verbal communication and self-expression easy, it is necessary to be patient and wait until they indicate by sound, eye movement, nod or small gesture that a need has been expressed or a choice made.[3] This can help the child feel empowered and in control of a situation. One should never assume that a child is deaf or unable to communicate and understand – it is important to focus on their ability and not their disability. The child should be given praise and encouragement for effort, not just achievement, and be told how well they are doing.[3] A source of frustration could be the inability to express food preferences, hunger or satiety until a simple communication method is developed.[2] The child may be given fewer choices than usual for their age and have a high degree of dependency on caregivers.

The child's ability to interact and control their environment should be incorporated into treatment programmes, and their likes and preferences acknowledged when planning a feeding regime. It is important to involve the child where possible in shopping for food and presenting meals attractively, and this will be useful in making the child an active partner in the preparation process.

Such an approach may help reinforce the child's unintentional signals such as eye, hand and body movements, thus teaching the child to give clearer signals of needs and wants.[1] Indications of preferences will subsequently be recognized and the child must then be offered choices, therefore learning that they have some control over the food they are offered.

Meals should be relaxed and in a family group so children learn a regular routine and observe eating as a source of pleasure. It is important to consider how some control can be given to the child and how the adult can limit intrusions of this control. For instance, the carer may allow some food that the child feeds themselves although this should not comprise the bulk of the meal. The family should try to eat at the same time, therefore minimizing the intense focus on the child's eating. Mealtimes, where possible, should be more of a playtime with the family, provided this does not become too much of a distraction.

If the child is unable to speak, they may benefit from augmentive communication in order to give clear signals. This should include signs and indicators in the form of electronic technology or use of a dedicated speech output device.

FEEDING INTERACTIONS

It is important to remember that we eat not simply for the purpose of maintenance of growth of our bodies but also as a fundamental social activity which we share with others.[1] Mealtimes should promote independence, even if it's messy, and they should be sociable and friendly with opportunities to interact and learn.[3] Social and verbal interaction is an important component of the eating process and it should be enjoyable for the child and carer.

Although it is important to promote independence in self-feeding, it is essential that the child's nutritional status is not compromised for the sake of independence.[6] Nutritional intake may be negatively affected by behavioural issues such as a short attention span or hyperactivity and these can be addressed by using smaller, more frequent meals. Diet should also be individualized to comply with religious and ethical considerations.[7]

PARENTS/CARERS

Consideration should also be given to meeting the psychological needs of the parent or carer through support. Mothers may feel unable to leave their disabled child in anyone else's care for fear they will be unable to cope at mealtimes. Difficulty feeding a child can impose severe restrictions on activities and opportunities for the mother both within and outside the home. These can be further complicated by negative feelings generated by the child's failure to thrive and inability to reward the mother by returning affection.[1]

Intervention programmes

It is important to remember that helping the carer is a way of helping the child. When devising a programme to address behavioural issues, it is important to follow these simple guidelines that aim to identify and address any specific needs:[1,4]

- get detailed information about what happens during a mealtime;
- identify aspects of the mealtime that the carer would like to change;
- identify factors that may be causing or contributing to the feeding problem;
- determine the reason the carer has sought the intervention;
- be clear about the objectives and goals for the child and carer;
- write a list of stressful things at mealtimes that can be tackled one at a time;
- introduce change slowly and in small stages and let the child adjust in a calm way;
- choose appropriate times to experiment with a change in routine;

- allow the child to make informed choices whenever possible and try and involve in planning the weekly menu;
- keep the carers' own feelings in perspective and reassure them that:
  - it is natural to feel discouraged if the child has not eaten after they have invested preparation time,
  - they may experience negative emotions which can promote boredom and apathy,
  - they should talk to other parents and seek help and advice.

Enteral nutrition: the practicalities

Disabled children with oral motor dysfunction and feeding difficulties frequently require adjunctive feeding methods. Enteral nutrition can be defined as the provision of liquid formula diets by mouth or tube directly into the gastrointestinal tract. The last two decades have seen rising interest in enteral nutrition and there are increasing numbers of children living in the community who require enteral tube feeding to achieve their optimal nutritional status.[8]

Consideration of a child for home enteral tube feeding should start with an assessment of family resources and individual needs that addresses issues such as coping methods for the level of care required.[2] The special needs of the child, family and carer should be identified and arrangements made to fulfil these needs in order to prepare them for the transfer of care from hospital to home. Home feeding programmes should be tailored to meet individual requirements and to cause minimal disruption to the child and carers lifestyle. Compromise may be necessary to adapt feeding regimes to suit individual lifestyles, while at the same time ensuring that the child receives adequate nutrition.[2] Programmes should involve the arranging and coordination of continuing care, whether this care is provided by the family, health care professionals, social services, education, voluntary bodies or a combination of them all.[2]

Types of enteral feeding tube

There are many types of equipment available on the market and it is important for the child and family to be aware of the options available to them and to be involved in choosing that which is most suitable. The choice of tube must be discussed with the family before a decision is made.[9] Table 5.1 sets out the specific details of tube use for the nasogastric tube, gastrostomy tube and jejunostomy feeding.[9]

Feeding regime

There are two feed delivery methods available for children who are being enterally fed: bolus and continuous. Certain situations dictate a preferred feeding regime but it is important to be flexible where possible so that the child and family can maintain their usual daily activities with minimal disruption to lifestyle and routine. Table 5.2 compares the two feeding regimes:[1,2]

Table 5.1 Nasogastric tube, gastrostomy tube and jejunostomy feeding[9]

	Nasogastric tube	Gastrostomy tube	Jejunostomy
Use	To bypass the oropharynx and deliver food directly into stomach	If tube feeding is required beyond 6 weeks, unsafe swallow or recurrent aspiration, oro-aversive behaviour, prolonged feeding times, compromised growth	To bypass any upper gastro-intestinal tract pathology
Indications	Functioning gastrointestinal tract but unable to meet requirements orally	As for nasogastric tube plus congenital abnormalities, long-term need, oesophageal injury, oesophageal dysmotility	Persistent vomiting, severe delayed gastric emptying, gastroparesis, uncontrolled gastro-oesophageal reflux, pulmonary aspiration
Advantages	Simplest, most obvious first choice that is relatively easily inserted	Long-term use, durable, aesthetically pleasing as can be changed to a low profile device	Can be nasal, trans-pyloric, trans-gastric placement or via surgical jejunostomy
Problems	Misplacement (trachea, small intestine), accidental removal, occlusion, body image, trauma/ulceration/perforation, dysphagia/nausea/oral/nasal phobia, difficulty confirming gastric placement of tube tip, discomfort	Large bowel perforation/fistula, peritonitis, accidental displacement leading to closure of stoma, infection, over granulation, occlusion, migration	Dumping syndrome, migration, displacement, perforation, tube occlusion. (Jejunostomy feeding should always be continuous – boluses can cause pain, diarrhoea and dumping syndrome)
Contra-indications	Persistent vomiting, severe delayed gastric emptying, intestinal obstruction, uncontrolled gastro-oesophageal reflux with risk of pulmonary aspiration	As for nasogastric tube plus gross ascites, severe obesity, clotting abnormalities, a ventriculo-peritoneal shunt is a relative contraindication	Complete intestinal obstruction, clotting abnormalities, gross ascites, severe obesity

Table 5.2 Bolus compared with continuous feeding[1,2]

	Bolus	Continuous
Advantages	Stimulates normal feeding patterns and encourages the secretion of gut hormones	Allows higher fluid intake with decreased risk of gastric distension and thus gastro-oesophageal reflux and aspiration
Disadvantages	Delayed gastric emptying, gastro-oesophageal reflux and vomiting, respiratory difficulty due to gastric distension	The patient is attached to the equipment for the duration of the feed
Delivery	Can be given 3–4 hourly throughout the day which physiologically mimics the normal feeding pattern and can be adapted to fit in with family meal times. These can be more time consuming but are preferred if feeding is required long term as it allows freedom and mobility	The stomach acts as a reservoir for food and regulates the amount delivered into the small intestine thus increasing tolerance. Nocturnal feeding can be used to supplement daytime intake with decreased inconvenience to parents and carers
Specific uses	This method is recommended if a fundoplication has been performed as it reduces the chance of large volumes accumulating in the stomach	Continuous feeds are essential if there is severe gastro-oesophageal reflux – should be used in conjunction with anti-reflux medications and positioning

Support

Meeting the nutritional requirements of children with neurological impairments takes a tremendous amount of time, energy and patience. Parents must be given adequate information regarding their child's condition and dietary needs with careful explanations and participation sessions.[7] Despite the distress and adverse consequences associated with oral feeding, contemplating gastrostomy tube insertion is not easy and many mothers feel that they have failed when the child is unable to eat orally.[10] Parents may often be against the idea of a gastrostomy at first and should be given all the information they need in order to make a decision. They should be given the opportunity to discuss ways that gastrostomy tube feeding may be delivered to determine which one is in the best interest of the child and fits in with the family routine.[11]

Decision-making

For the child with impaired decision-making capacity, it is the parents or family members who are responsible for making treatment decisions. Medical treatment decisions are often complex and the choice has to be made between two alternatives, both of which may generate undesirable outcomes. Many decisions are about interventions that could cause suffering, involve extra financial burden and disrupt bodily integrity.[10] There are four main factors which contribute to uncertainty concerning decision-making, and which should be addressed when dealing with families faced with this choice:[10]

- lack of information;
- social pressure, and pressure from medical team;
- lack of support;
- lack of clarity about personal opinions regarding value trade offs.

Professionals and families must learn from each other in order to work as a collaborative team when making health care decisions.[12] Information should be given to the family prior to the decision-making process and both the advantages and disadvantages of the procedure explained in full.[10] Where possible, carers should be given the opportunity to talk to other families who have been through the same decision-making process as this has been found to be of great help and normalizes the issues and concerns.[10,13]

The perceived pressures regarding feeding tube insertion are both for and against the surgery. Some medical professionals may regard the tube as unnecessary, and people in the support network such as family members, or respite carers, may refuse to care for the child with a feeding tube in place.[10]

Concerns regarding the value trade offs of feeding tube insertion do not just revolve around the medical or practical aspects but also how it will impact on everyday lives.[14] There is a perception among families that the child's global abnormality is emphasized by the placement of a feeding tube, and that their disability becomes more visible to those around them.[12] It is important for the family to feel that they are balancing their needs as a whole by maintaining a sense of normality in parity with the need for improved health and nutrition.[12] Reassurance should be given that tube feeding will not deprive the child of the pleasure and socialization of eating, and that the nurturance provided through the process of orally feeding their child can still be provided as an adjunct to tube feeds.[10,12]

Carers should be given the opportunity to discuss any concerns with the medical team, and be given written information to take home. This allows for discussion with their family and friends, and for an informed choice to be made in a supportive, familiar environment.

Support sources

There are day to day obstacles that confront paediatric patients and their families who are enterally fed. Support for the carer, and the child who is enterally fed, can come from many sources and may include parent, carer, siblings, relatives, friends, respite, health and social professionals.

It is, however, the parent or carer who takes day to day responsibility for the management of tube feeding. This can be divided into three main areas:[8]

- practical management: administering feeds, cleaning the stoma site, flushing tubes, maintaining intake;
- social management: obtaining support from social services, access to education, going out to restaurants, and going on holiday. Coping with social situations (meals etc.);
- emotional management: coping with their own feelings of guilt and anger, other peoples reactions etc.

Families need support for all three management issues, and the nurse is ideally placed to take on this role as they are experts in the management of tube feeds and can provide telephone guidance to the family. The nurse can work in partnership with the family by listening to their concerns and recognizing, and maximizing, the family's expertise.[14] These three issues can greatly affect family functioning, social life, finances, employment, cognition, depression, anxiety and pain control. Some parents can off-set negative issues such as stigma and sleepless nights against new found benefits that the family experience, such as more time spent together and less pressure at mealtimes.[8] A great source of support for families new to the situation is contact with other families who have been through similar situations. This enables them to share their experiences with others who understand their concerns, which in turn may normalize the problems and decrease feelings of isolation.[13] Web-based resources are becoming more popular and increasingly accessible: a selection of support sources can be found in Appendix 2.

Intervention planning

Once the decision has been made to place an enteral feeding tube in a child, there is extensive groundwork and planning required to help prepare the child and carers.[4] Previous experience has highlighted those areas where carers feel they need most support[15] and these include:

- information about the effect of tube feeding on the child and family;
- support to deal with problems arising from care of the tube fed child;
- problems with the supply of equipment and feeds after discharge from hospital;
- coordination of support services.

Knowledge of these factors can act as a guide to improve the service offered to patients after discharge from hospital.

Assessment
Before tube feeding commences, the child needs to have a multidisciplinary nutritional, physical and psychological assessment. This will help establish that tube feeding is an appropriate intervention and identifies the most beneficial method of administration. The child, parents and carers should be involved in all decisions relating to care and they should be included in discussions of all aspects of practical, social and emotional management of tube feeding. Including them in these discussions will promote understanding of the reasons for the intervention and improve treatment compliance.

Planning and coordination
Parents, carers and, as far as is possible the child, must understand the need for tube feeding and must be competent and confident to undertake the procedures taught. This ensures safety for the child and family and checks they can demonstrate safe techniques, recognize problems if they arise and know what action to take. Education should begin on the ward as an integral part of the discharge planning process and the community nurse should visit to provide support in providing a suitable environment for tube feeds, such as safe storage and infection control. Families should first observe procedures, and then carry them out under supervision while being assessed for competency. Any verbal information given should also be supported by written guidelines reinforcing the same information and in a language they can understand.

Preparation for the procedure
As with all children, toys are a very helpful tool when preparing for procedures. Young children are naturally curious and eager to explore and investigate their environment to discover how things work. This is done through play, although the child with special needs may not always show this natural curiosity. This does not mean that that they are not interested in playing or cannot play, but it does mean that they may need more encouragement and help to become involved.[3] For the child who is visually impaired, the toy or teaching aid should be placed in their hands. The child should be given help to move their fingers over the object as explanations are given so that they can understand its shape, texture and purpose.[3]
There tends to be a heavy bias of support and training aids towards English language versions. The UK is a multicultural, multiracial, multifaith, multilingual society and effective training programmes should be developed with interpreters for all of the appropriate languages.[2]

Any home nutrition programmes should be designed to ensure that the child and family are equal partners in care and family are equal participants in all discussions.[2]

Preparation for tube feeds
Psychological preparation of the child and family pre- and post-feeding is essential and an experienced play specialist can provide invaluable support. Imaginative, interactive

training aids should be used, such as videos, dummies, computer training, written and pictorial guidelines.[9]

Detailed preparation of families takes time. The passing of a nasogastric tube or insertion of a gastrostomy can be a distressing time for parents, carers and children. The child should be prepared as for a painful procedure, and followed up sensitively according to their needs. The key areas likely to cause distress should be identified and a frank discussion should take place about the degree of discomfort expected. Feedback between the hospital and community team is essential in order to facilitate the smooth transfer between services.

Equipment and supplies

The child who is due to receive tube feeds in the community should have their home environment assessed in order to address any difficulties, and plan for discharge in advance. They should have all the necessary equipment and supplies at home and parents should know how, who, when and where to contact to obtain supplies. It is easier if there is one specific individual in the community who can be identified as a contact point for the discharge process and ongoing care, and a referral made prior to discharge. Any information taught or given to the family should be shared with the multidisciplinary team in the community. It is important to document all requirements (type of feed, amount, method, regime and equipment) and provide information to the relevant community team. The family doctor should be contacted where necessary to provide a prescription for the feed, and supplies for home delivery should be ordered in advance with 7 days supply given from hospital. Single use items should not be re-used and clinical waste disposed of appropriately.

School

If the child receives feeds at school, or attends with a feeding tube in situ, guidelines should be provided for administration and staff should receive the necessary training and assessment (storage of feed, cleaning equipment, infection control and risk assessment). Guidelines should be provided for emergency procedures should the tube fall out and need replacing, and supplies of extra feed delivered to school if necessary. See Appendix 3 for an example of universal guidelines. The team should promote inclusion of the child within the school environment and avoid disruption to their normal routine.

Holistic development

All aspects of the child's physical, social and emotional development should be promoted. Tube feeding can be planned to fit in with normal lifestyle and should not limit social and emotional development. It is important to promote social inclusion and minimize the disruption that receiving tube feeds may cause. Consideration should be given to the child's physical appearance, such as the way a nasogastric tube is taped which should be done after discussion to find out the child's preferences. Oral stimulation (age appropriate) should be encouraged during feeds to promote the association of sucking or eating with the sensation of feeding and satiety.

The tube fed child should be fed at the meal table and encouraged to use utensils, therefore encouraging normal socialization with feeding and meals. Tube fed children should also be encouraged to eat, if it is safe for them to have an oral diet, and encouraged to use their mouth in play (blowing, kissing, touching their mouth). It is important to provide ongoing support to maintain and improve their dietary intake where appropriate and the tube should be considered as a supplement to a normal diet where possible. Encouragement can help children enjoy the taste and feel of food and enable families to maintain the social and psychological bonds that mealtimes allow.

Follow-up

All children on enteral feeds should have a regular multidisciplinary team review as their needs will vary according to their stage of physical, social and emotional development and underlying medical needs. The assessment should include measurements of weight, height, head circumference, mid-upper arm circumference and skin fold thickness (where possible) (see Chapter 2). Details should be recorded of their oral intake, feed type, feeding regime, equipment used and supplies. The multidisciplinary team should monitor the practical, social and emotional impact of feeds on the family as a whole as the impact of tube feeding on the family is often overlooked or grossly underestimated.[2]

For some children embarking on feeding via enteral tubes, serious and unintended social deprivations may result. We eat for many reasons other than providing nourishment and the child who is tube fed may have less access or be excluded from the social opportunities that accompany eating.[4] We eat for companionship, celebration, ritual and comfort, and mealtimes provide an opportunity for family integration while at the same time giving rhythm and regulation to ones day.[4] Social situations such as eating out or going on holiday may be affected by tube feeding because of inconvenience or public ignorance.[13] These factors all have important implications for health, social care and education professionals and should be considered when caring for a child who is tube fed.

Training

Training given to parents regarding enteral tube feeding should be carried out by trained professionals. They should be able to discuss the social, emotional and mechanical aspects of feeding and provide verbal and written information.[9] As discussed above carers and parents should be assessed for their ability to undertake all procedures without supervision.[16] This should include school and respite carers, and guidelines should be produced for all those involved in the care of the child to allow for consistent, fair and safe practice.[8] These should comply with local guidelines and policy and adhere to best practice guides (see Appendix 3). It is also very important to put families in contact with other parents about their experiences.

Discharge planning
Discharge planning and carer training in all aspects of tube feeding should be one of the key aspects of hospital care prior to discharge.[2]

Teaching home enteral nutrition should involve programmes of care based on detailed assessment, planning, implementation and evaluation of the patient. The approach to training should have its focus on family-centred care with the parents working in full partnership with the health professionals. It is important to be aware that children have specific physical, social, psychological and physiological needs both at home and in school or respite. In both the education of parents and in the production of carer guidelines meticulous attention to detail is required (see Appendix 3).

Detailed information should be given to the carers about the necessity for tube feeds and the likely duration. Factors that should be taken into account when training carers/parents are outlined below: [2,16]

- psychological preparation:
  - reasons for enteral feeding,
  - how the tube is inserted and how long it will be in place,
  - emotional and psychosocial implications,
  - social and practical implications for the child and carer,
  - play therapist to support preparation of child,
  - visual aids such as booklets, videos and dummies should be used;
- Safety:
  - explanation of anatomy related to gastrointestinal/respiratory tract,
  - complications of tube placement,
  - microbiological contamination of feed;
- oral stimulation:
  - written information on the importance of ongoing input,
  - referral to speech and language therapist;
- community:
  - staff contacts given for hospital and community,
  - support groups (see Appendix 2);
- hygiene:
  - reasons for hand washing,
  - microbiological issues for consideration,
  - hand washing technique,
  - decontamination of work surfaces for feed preparation;
- feed preparation:
  - parents should be confident in preparation of feed,

  - understand feed components,
  - decanting and storage;
- equipment:
  - familiarization of pump and equipment,
  - alarm systems identified,
  - running set through,
  - storing equipment,
  - contacts for supplies;
- tube care:
  - care of tube,
  - checking position,
  - tube replacement/tube change,
  - aspiration technique and safety,
  - flushing tube,
  - tube rotation,
  - unblocking the tube,
  - skin care;
- feeds:
  - the consistency and amount of oral feeds will be determined by the dietitian,
  - type, volume and times of feed,
  - administration of food and drugs,
  - fluid requirements and recognition of signs of dehydration or fluid overload,
  - contacts for supplies;
- common problems and solutions:
  - what to do in an emergency;
  - notify parents immediately if any changes with feeding plan.

It is important to remember that any information given to the family or carers may have to be provided in other languages and that it is accessible for those with difficulty with written information.

Health promotion

Risk management should be seen as an integral part of health care, ensuring the provision of a high quality, safe service to patients.[16] Health care workers should practice universal precautions when dealing with bodily fluids, and this practice taught to carers of children receiving enteral feeds at home. Carers are not required to wear protective clothing but must be made aware that the risks of bacterial contamination of enteral feeds and the possible risk of infection around the gastrostomy site can lead to complications.[16] Poor handling is the main cause of bacterial contamination of sterile enteral feeds and by reducing the risk of infection from this cause the incidence of morbidity and mortality in health care can be reduced.[16] Feed contamination is common in the home and can lead to gastroenteritis.[2] The main sources of contamination are outlined in Table 5.3.[16]

It is not possible to eliminate all incidents of microbial contamination of enteral tube feeds, but everyone involved in home enteral tube feeding has a role to play in trying to decrease the risk.[17]

Table 5.3 The main sources of feed contamination[16]

Problem	Cause	Solution
Touch contamination of equipment	Poor technique and manipulation of the feed system	Select feeding systems that require: Least amount of handling Minimum number of connections Well-designed connectors
Contaminated feed	Use of non-sterile ingredients Reconstitution of powdered feeds Decanting Excessive handling Inappropriate storage Container damage Excessive hanging time (Not longer than 24 hours if sterile, 4 hours if not)	Use sterile liquid feeds where possible Provide adequate teaching on hygiene, and safe handling and storage of all feeds
Contaminated additives such as medications, flush solutions, supplements	Misuse of equipment such as prolonged or re-use of feeding sets, syringes or connectors	Freshly opened sterile water to be used for dilution, reconstitution and flushing. Single-use items to be disposed of appropriately
Cross-infection	Failure to adequately decontaminate hands or equipment between feeds	Adequate teaching required on: Hand washing technique Prep surface decontamination Sterilisation of equipment
Site problems: colonization or infection of percutaneous endoscopic gastrostomy site	Poor hand hygiene technique	Cuts and sores on hands must be covered with waterproof dressing Feeds and tubes shouldn't be handled if skin infections or diarrhoea and vomiting present

Dental health

For the child with neurological impairments, the diversity of their condition means their health may be affected in ways that has implications for dental care.[18] Dental problems may both contribute to and be an outcome of poor nutrition and dental caries, periodontal disease and gingival hyperplasia can all contribute to feeding difficulties in their own right.[1,7] Secondary orthodontic problems may also occur as a consequence of oral motor mal-development and could include malocclusion, overbite and overjet.[1] Table 5.4 outlines some of the common dental problems experienced by children with neurological impairments: [2,7,18]

Children with neurological impairments require oral hygiene to be carried out with the correct and adequate equipment. Information can be provided by occupational

Table 5.4 Common dental problems experienced by children with neurological impairments [2,7,18]

Problem	Cause	Consequences
Inability/ difficulty cleaning teeth and having dental care	Physical limitations, oral hypersensitivity, lack of cooperation, fear	Increases the risk of gum disease and leads to a build up of harmful bacteria which may cause bad breath and affect general health
Abnormal neuromuscular coordination of the tongue, lips and cheeks	Lack of normal chewing and tongue movements to move food around mouth and clear food from teeth	Poor dental alignment, gum disease and tissue problems
Damaging oral habits	Bruxism, rumination, pouching and pica	May wear teeth down to the gum over a period of time, pain
Behavioural problems	Inability to communicate toothache or other sensations	Self-injury such as tongue, cheek and lip biting, finger, arm and hand chewing
Poor enamel formation	Gastro-oesophageal reflux which causes dental erosion and loss of tooth structure. Tooth grinding Acidic drinks, sugary medications	May cause increased sensitivity, pain, dental caries, tooth loss
Dry mouth, gingival hyperplasia	Drug side effects from tricyclic antidepressants, phenytoin and phenobarbital	May be irritating and increase dental problems by adversely affecting dental hygiene and causing impaired chewing

therapists, and speech and language therapists, who can advise on the correct equipment, positioning and therapeutic techniques to assist with good oral hygiene. Children should also be registered with a paediatric dentist with experience of children with oral and behavioural difficulties, who should be consulted for regular dental checks. Dental visits should start by 1 year of age, or within 6 months of the first tooth.[18] The community dental service should be able to recommend such a dentist.[15]

Caregivers should be educated on the appropriate methods of preventive dental practices, and teaching should be given on the following aspects:[2,6,18]

- fresh fruit and vegetables should be offered, where appropriate, for the food texture;
- frequent brushing promoted (at least twice per day). Electric tooth brushing may be used which could introduce an aspect of novelty;
- fluoride is essential and can be found as toothpaste, mouth rinses, brush-on gels, drops and tablets (as recommended by a dentist);
- fissure sealing;
- prevention of trauma;
- prevention of tooth wear – including effective treatment of GOR and vomiting;
- acidic and sugary snacks, drinks and medications should be discouraged;
- get child used to touching gums etc. from before they have teeth;
- lots of praise for positive oral hygiene practices.

Promoting the dental health of disabled children must be considered as an important component of multidisciplinary care.[1] Unresolved dental problems often have a negative impact on food intake, as well as health and quality of life.[6]

Conclusion

The role of the multidisciplinary team in caring for the nutritional needs of the child with neurological impairment and their family is multifaceted. With many disciplines converging to achieve a unified goal, the need for efficient communication and coordination of services is paramount. Implementing the various strategies and solutions that have been put forward requires clear objectives established at the outset for the child, carers and team.

References

1. Sullivan PB, Rosenbloom L. *Feeding the Disabled Child.* London: MacKeith Press, 1996.
2. Holden C, MacDonald A. *Nutrition and Child Health.* London: Harcourt Publishers, 2000.
3. Dare A, O'Donovan M. *Good Practice in Caring For Young Children with Special Needs,* 2nd edn. Cheltenham: Nelson thornes, 2002.
4. Crane S. Feeding the handicapped child – a review of intervention strategies. *Nutr Health* 1987; 5: 109–18.

5. Craig GM, Scambler G. Negotiating mothering against the odds: gastrostomy tube feeding, stigma, governmentality and disabled children. *Soc Sci Med* 2006; **62**: 1115–25.
6. Ekvall SW, Ekvall VK. *Pediatric Nutrition in Chronic Diseases and Developmental Disorders*, 2nd edn. New York: Oxford University Press, 2005.
7. Suskind RM, Lewinter-Suskind L. *Textbook of Pediatric Nutrition*, 2nd edn. New York: Raven Press, 1993.
8. Townsley R, Robinson C. *Effective Support Services to Disabled Children who are Tube Fed*. Bristol: University of Bristol, 1997.
9. Holden C, MacDonald A. An overview of paediatric feeding. *Clin Nutr* 2003; **7**: 3–4.
10. Guerriere DN, McKeever P, Llewellyn-Thomas H, Berall G. Mothers' decisions about gastrostomy tube insertion in children: factors contributing to uncertainty. *Dev Med Child Neurol* 2003; **45**: 470–6.
11. Carter C. *Enteral Feeding in Children with Severe Cerebral Palsy*. Trowbridge: SHS Nutricia, 2006.
12. Brotherson MJ, Oakland MJ, Secrist-Mertz C, Lichfield R, Larson K. Quality of life issues for families who make the decision to use a feeding tube for their child with disabilities. *J Assoc Pers Sev Handicaps* 1995; **20**: 202–12.
13. Michaelis CA, Warzak WJ, Stanek K, Van RC. Parental and professional perceptions of problems associated with long-term pediatric home tube feeding. *J Am Diet Assoc* 1992; **92**: 1235–8.
14. Sleigh G. Mothers' voice: a qualitative study on feeding children with cerebral palsy. *Child Care Health Dev* 2005; **31**: 373–83.
15. Moss D. *Nasogastric and Gastrostomy Tube Feeding for Children being Cared for in the Community. Best Practice Statement.* Edinburgh: NHS Quality Improvement Scotland, 2003.
16. Skipper L, Cuffling J, Pratelli N. *Enteral Feeding. Infection Control Guidelines*. London: Infection Control Nurses Association, 2003.
17. Anderton A. *Microbial Contamination of Enteral Tube Feeds*. Trowbridge: Nutricia, 2000
18. Scope. *Dental Care for People with Cerebral Palsy*. London: SCOPE, 2007 Available from: www.scope.org.uk/downloads/factsheets/word/dental.doc

Chapter 6

Gastrointestinal Disorders: Assessment and management

Peter B Sullivan

The enteric nervous system

The enteric nervous system may contain as many as one billion neurons: 1% of the number of neurons in the brain, and considerably more than the number of neurons in the spinal cord. The activity of this enteric nervous system is modulated by inputs from the central nervous system. Modulation of the neural activity in the enteric nervous system by extrinsic innervation is abnormal in many children with central nervous system disorders. Thus, it is not surprising that insults to the brain may result in significant dysfunction in the gastrointestinal tract.

Foregut dysmotility

This gastrointestinal dysfunction manifests primarily, but not exclusively, as a dysmotility in the foregut. The foregut starts at the mouth and ends in the second part of the duodenum and is most severely affected because of it great density of extrinsic innervations. These arise either from the spine via prevertebral ganglia (spinal arc) or directly from the medulla in the two-way traffic in the vagus nerve. Break down in efferent control is associated ultimately with electromechanical disassociation leading to abnormal motility and symptoms.

Oral motor impairment

Symptoms from oral motor impairment include feeding problems, drooling and gagging as well as dysarthria. Uncoordinated swallowing increases the risk of pulmonary aspiration which may or may not be heralded by recurrent coughing and choking with feeds. Those children with the severest general motor deficit (bilateral cerebral palsy) are, as might be expected, also those with the most severe degree of oral motor impairment. This is because development of oral motor skills mirrors general neurological maturation. This development requires the coordination of the movement of a total of 31 pairs of striated muscles in the mouth, pharynx and oesophagus by 6 cranial nerves, the brain stem and the cerebral cortex. When the central control of this mass of musculature is severely impaired there is little chance of getting sufficient quantities of food and drink safely into the oesophagus.

Oesophageal dysmotility

Once in the oesophagus the smooth passage of the swallowed bolus may be disrupted as a result of dysmotile peristalsis. Manometric studies in children with 'psychomotor retardation' have revealed incomplete relaxation of the upper oesophageal sphincter and significantly decreased amplitude of peristaltic waves in the oesophagus.[1] A significant decrease in the pressure in the lower oesophageal sphincter accompanies these abnormalities and this 'failure' of the lower oesophageal sphincter is probably the main reason for the high prevalence of gastro-oesophageal reflux (GOR) in children with neurological impairment.

Gastro-oesophageal reflux (GOR)

The high incidence of GOR (15–75%) in children with neurological impairments is well-recognized. Several reasons have been proposed to account for this high incidence in children with cerebral palsy including hiatus hernia, adoption of a prolonged supine position, and increased intra-abdominal pressure secondary to spasticity, scoliosis or seizures. Nevertheless, central nervous system dysfunction is likely to be the prime cause of GOR. As a result of neuromuscular incoordination, the anti-reflux function of the lower oesophageal sphincter mechanism and oesophageal motility are significantly impaired. Dysmotility in the stomach (see below) also predisposes towards GOR. Thus food and digestive factors such as acid and pepsin reflux rostrally from the stomach into the oesophagus. They may reflux back as far as the pharynx which, in those with an impaired ability to protect the larynx, can lead to pulmonary aspiration (see below). Moreover, as shown by combined manometric and pH studies in the lower oesophagus, the associated oesophageal dysmotility reduces the effectiveness of acid and pepsin clearance from the oesophageal mucosa following GOR.[1] Thus the risk of peptic oesophagitis and gastro-oesophageal reflux disease (GORD) is enhanced.

Gastro-oesophageal reflux disease (GORD)

Chronic peptic oesophagitis may progress to oesophageal mucosal ulceration and stricture formation. Peptic oesophagitis is more likely to become a chronic symptom in children with neurological impairment. It is ironic that the learning deficit that usually accompanies neurological impairment also impairs the ability of the affected individual to communicate the main symptom of GORD which is pain. The burning epigastric pain articulated by affected individuals without neurological impairment that arises from peptic oesophagitis may be quite severe. In children with cerebral palsy the chronic dysphagia arising from GORD may be confused with behavioural food avoidance or aversion. Food related behaviour problems and rumination are common and found in about 40% of children with GORD and so should also prompt a search for GOR in children with neurological impairment. Alternatively, the discomfort from peptic oesophagitis may manifest itself in chronic irritability and crying or, much more rarely, as dystonic movements of the face and neck. In children with neurological impairment the objective hallmark of GORD is recurrent vomiting which occurs in over 80% of cases and which may further compromise their already precarious nutritional state. Vomiting, haematemesis, anaemia, rumination and regurgitation are all more common in individuals with neurological impairment who are suspected of having GORD than in those in whom GORD is not suspected.

Dental problems are an under recognized consequence of GOR; children with cerebral palsy have an increased prevalence of tooth erosion, which has been attributed to the presence of GOR. The investigation of GORD is described in Chapter 7.

Respiratory consequences of GORD
The association between GORD and respiratory complications (apnea, laryngitis, asthma/wheezing, chronic cough, chronic pulmonary aspiration, recurrent pneumonia and progressive lung injury) has been recognized for decades. In children with cerebral palsy poor nutritional status, ineffective cough and poor pulmonary reserve (due to chest wall deformity) increase the risk of significant morbidity and mortality from respiratory infections.

Antroduodenal dysmotility

Antroduodenal dysmotility contributes to GOR and is another component of foregut dysmotility in cerebral palsy. In healthy individuals, lower oesophageal sphincter contraction is provoked by distension of the gastric wall, through a vago–vagal reflex. This reflex arc involves the solitary tract nucleus, where the swallowing centre is located, and GOR may result from the lesions directly in the tegmentum of the medulla oblongata or from lesions in cortical areas that modulate brain stem activity. Vagal nerve dysfunction causes a relaxation of the proximal stomach and retroperistalsis secondary to inhibition of the gastric pacemaker. Antroduodenal motility studies have revealed absent spontaneous fasting migrating motor complexes and postprandial hypomotility.[2] Electrogastrography has revealed a variety of gastric dysrhythmias including both bradygastria and tachygastria. Thus, gastroduodenal dysrhythmia and electromechanical uncoupling lead to distension of the fundus of the stomach which in turn promotes transient relaxation of the lower oesophageal sphincter and GOR. This electromechanical uncoupling may also be associated with delayed gastric emptying.

Delayed gastric emptying

Delayed gastric emptying accompanies some (28–50%) cases of GOR. Delayed gastric emptying has been demonstrated in both healthy children and those with disorders of the central nervous system. Children with delayed gastric emptying are more at risk of developing gas bloat and persistent retching after fundoplication. Del Giudice et al reported that 67% of children with cerebral palsy and GOR had delayed gastric emptying.[3] This association, however, may to some extent depend upon the type of food given. Nevertheless, trying to treat GOR without effectively treating delayed gastric emptying, may be one of the reasons why both conservative and surgical treatment of GOR in profoundly disabled children gives such poor results.[4] Opinions have differed, however, as to whether or not a pyloroplasty should be performed at the same time as a fundoplication; Fonkalsrud et al[5] recommended pyloroplasty for patients with delayed gastric emptying, whereas Maxson et al found no clinical advantage from pyloroplasty.[6] This equivocal situation notwithstanding, there maybe a place for pyloroplasty in a few selected patients with objective evidence of delayed gastric emptying and persistent symptoms attributable to this, although the risk of precipitating the dumping syndrome has to be borne in mind.

The dumping syndrome

The dumping syndrome is a group of symptoms that occur when food or liquid enters the small intestine too rapidly. Common symptoms of dumping are refusal to eat, postprandial nausea, retching, tachycardia, paleness and lethargy and watery diarrhoea. Dumping syndrome is also common following a Nissen fundoplication in children. A Nissen fundoplication increases intragastric pressure and also increases gastric emptying, particularly if a pyloroplasty has been performed. Together with impaired vagal reflexes, this leads to rapid delivery of undigested hyperosmolar chyme into the proximal gut, which promotes fluid shifts into the bowel and the sudden increase in intestinal blood flow results in a decreasing circulating blood volume and a brisk intake in atrial natriuretic peptide and activation of the renin–aldosterone axis. This pathophysiological process correlates with abdominal discomfort, vasomotor symptoms and tachycardia. Rapid gastrointestinal passage of chyme exceeds the digestive and absorptive capacity of the small intestine and the food reaches the distal gut, leading to supraphysiological release of several gut hormones. The treatment of the dumping syndrome is to inhibit rapid gastric emptying and the postcibal reactive hypoglycemia and, therefore, readily absorbable mono-disaccharide and polymers should be replaced by complex carbohydrates, including uncooked starch. If this fails, continuous intragastric feeding may be necessary.

Retching

Retching refers to the laboured rhythmic activity of the diaphragm and anterior abdominal wall musculature which precedes vomiting and is the first part of the emetic reflex. It is important to realize that vomiting in children with neurological impairment is not always caused by GOR and that activation of the emetic reflex is another important mechanism. The sensory and motor pathways of the vagus nerve, the area postrema and the nuclei of the vagus nerve play a major role in the emetic reflex. Gastric vagal afferents are potent activators of the emetic reflex and it is possible that in some children with neurodevelopmental disability the emetic reflex is hypersensitive or there may be loss of its physiological inhibition. Such emesis is characterized by a prodrome of salivation, tachycardia, peripheral vasoconstriction, nausea and retching and, in contrast with the relatively effortless vomiting associated with GOR, it is forceful. Vomiting accompanied by retching is seen more often in children with neurodevelopmental disability than in children without such disability and when this occurs preoperatively they are three times more likely to retch following fundoplication than non-retchers.[7] Retching post-fundoplication may drive the wrap at the gastro-oesophageal junction through the diaphragmatic hiatus and be associated with failure of the fundal wrap.[8]

Management of GORD

The medical treatment of GORD

The advent of proton pump inhibitors (PPI) for use in children has had a very significant impact on the treatment of gastro-oesophageal reflux disease. Moreover, in some centres, this has been associated with a dramatic decrease in the number of surgical anti-reflux procedures performed in children.[9] Nevertheless, the evidence base for medical treatment of gastro-oesophageal reflux in this group of children is confused because systematic studies of the role of proton pump inhibitors in treating gastro-oesophageal reflux have tended to be exclusive of children with neurological impairment, because such data complicate the analysis. Vomiting usually persists despite PPI therapy, although a reduction in vomiting in children with neurological impairment treated with PPI is not infrequently observed. Proton pump inhibitors are superior to Histamine type 2 receptor antagonists (H2RA) as they reduce meal induced acid secretion which H2RAs do not. Administration of baclofen has been shown to reduce the frequency of vomiting and the total number of acid refluxes in children with neurological impairment with GORD. There is no prokinetic drug currently on the market that has been demonstrated to be uniformly effective in the treatment of gastro-oesophageal reflux disease and, although domperidone is widely prescribed, a recent systematic review failed to provide objective evidence of its efficacy for the treatment of gastro-oesophageal reflux in children.[10] It is commonly found that response to conventional medical therapy is poor and anti-reflux surgery is frequently required, especially when gastrostomy tube feeding is also needed for nutrition.

The surgical treatment of GORD

The surgical anti-reflux procedure that is most commonly performed is the Nissen fundoplication and less often the Thal procedure. Laparoscopic fundoplication can also be performed safely and with equivalent results in children with neurological impairment. Irrespective of the surgical technique employed fundoplication is associated with higher morbidity and mortality rates in children with neurological impairment, as compared with children without such impairment.[11] Following standard Nissen fundoplication, postoperative morbidity rates of up to 50% and re-operation rates of up to 20% and mortality rates up to 50% are quoted.[12] Major complications can occur intra- and postoperatively including hepatic vein laceration, bowel perforation, tension pneumothorax, paraoesophageal hernia and small bowel obstruction. Children with neurological impairment have more than twice the complication rate, three times the morbidity rate and four times the anti-reflux re-operation rate than children without neurological impairment. No single symptom is reliably predictive of recurrent gastro-oesophageal reflux.

Recurrent gastro-oesophageal reflux often leads to a second operation but re-do fundoplications fare no better with a failure rate of up to 28% quoted. It is necessary to have a high index of suspicion for the development of recurrent gastrooesophageal reflux after anti-reflux procedures in children with neurological impairment and to have a low threshold for proceeding to upper gastrointestinal contrast study and lower oesophageal pH study or endoscopy, to investigate this possibility (See Chapter 7).

Authors who study complications following fundoplication in their institutions report that this experience raises their threshold for performing this operation in children with neurological impairment.[4]

As noted by Smith et al back in 1992 'The use of fundoplication to improve outcome with an acceptably low risk does not appear to have been established'; this remains the situation 17 years later.[4] Some light on the mechanisms behind these poor results has arisen recently from studies in fundoplicated ferrets that have demonstrated the serosal fibrosis that occurs in the region of the wrap and in close proximity to the vagal nerve.[13] The extent to which these histological changes contribute to postoperative symptoms such as retching and dysphagia is not yet clear.

Alternative anti-reflux procedures

Alternatives to fundoplication include insertion of a gastrojejunal tube when gastrostomy is required or laparoscopic-assisted jejunostomy for enteral feeding in children with neurodevelopmental disability. Gastrojejunal tubes can be placed by interventional radiology or by the percutaneous route. There is possibly a greater risk of gastrojejunal intussusception and an adhesive small bowel obstruction with radiologically placed gastrojejunal tubes. Such procedures are probably no better than the standard technique, moreover, they do not treat gastro-oesophageal reflux, thus necessitating long-term medical treatment. Furthermore, jejunal feeding needs to be administered continuously by pump over most of the day.

An alternative operation, total oesophagogastric disconnection, has been reported in over 50 children. This operation, in which the gastro-oesophageal junction is transected and a Roux-en-Y loop of jejunum fashioned to the transected distal oesophagus, has been created as a result of a search for an alternative operation to the Nissen fundoplication, which would definitely prevent gastro-oesophageal reflux while at the same time allowing bolus feeds via the gastrostomy. Nevertheless, this is a procedure with a very high complication rate, 30% early complications and 41% late complications including small bowel obstruction, pancreatitis, pneumonia, paraoesophageal hernia. Some authors are very enthusiastic about this procedure and consider it to be the primary procedure for nutritional rehabilitation in children with neurological impairment. However, the majority view is that the high morbidity and the high mortality associated with oesophagogastric disconnection limit this procedure to a last ditch stand to rescue those children with neurological impairment and repeatedly failed Nissen fundoplications.

Gastrostomy tube feeding

Indications and technique

The feeding problems encountered in children with oral motor impairment and cerebral palsy and their associated nutritional and growth consequences are remediable to some extent by gastrostomy tube feeding. The indications for gastrostomy feeding in children with neurological impairment are shown in Box 6.1.

A gastrostomy feeding tube may be placed:

1. directly at either laparotomy or laparoscopy especially when an anti-reflux procedure is also indicated; or, more usually,
2. percutaneously by fibreoptic endoscope (percutaneous endoscopic gastrostomy, PEG).

It is usual practice to replace the gastrostomy tube by a skin-flush button device once the fistulous tract between the stomach and the anterior abdominal wall has consolidated after about 12 weeks. Preoperative assessment is mandatory before proceeding to PEG. Respiratory function should be evaluated and, if indicated, chest physiotherapy and appropriate antibiotics should be administered. It is particularly important to recognize significant GOR and prolonged lower oesophageal pH monitoring is routinely performed prior to gastrostomy insertion to determine the need for a surgical anti-reflux procedure. Previous recommendations that a 'protective' anti-reflux procedure should be performed in children with neurological impairment undergoing gastrostomy tube insertion have been challenged.[14,15]

Box 6.1 Indications for insertion of a gastrostomy feeding tube in children with neurological impairment

Insertion of a gastrostomy feeding tube is an increasingly common intervention in neurologically impaired children who:

- have an unsafe swallow;
- are unable to maintain a satisfactory nutritional state by oral feeding alone;
- have an inordinately long (>3 hours per day) oral feeding time;
- are dependant on nasogastric tube feeding.

Outcome

Gastrostomy tube feeding has been shown to lead to improved weight gain, reduced feeding time and improved quality of life for carers.[16]

Despite this evidence for efficacy the decision for caregivers regarding the insertion of a gastrostomy tube can be a difficult one with debate as to whether the benefits outweigh the risks. Previous qualitative studies have revealed that the concept of gastrostomy feeding has multiple and different meanings for caregivers. Common interpretations of the suggestion to implement gastrostomy tube feeding include 'giving up hope', 'relinquishing normal' or 'maternal failure' whereas others welcome the 'end of a struggle'. Paradoxically, the enhanced efficiency of feeding and the improvement in nutritional state following gastrostomy tube placement are well recognized in clinical practice to be associated with an ease in burden of the caregiver. Generally, the impact of gastrostomy feeding is positive, and many parents report that they wish the intervention had taken placer earlier. Smith and colleagues (1999) evaluated 45 families by semi-structured interview and found that 90% were pleased with the effect of tube feeding on their child and family life.[14] Negative reports may be associated with increased stress related to feeding or the presence of complications of gastrostomy tube feeding.

Complications

Complications of gastrostomy feeding have been described in 4–26% of cases. Major complications occur during or shortly after PEG insertion and include the risk from anaesthesia, laceration of the oesophagus, pneumoperitoneum, peritonitis and colonic perforation with the risk of colo-gastric fistula formation. Minor complications such as stoma leakage, cellulitis, and granulation tissue formation around the site of PEG insertion usually occur at a later stage. A number of case studies have reported that GOR worsened following gastrostomy feeding.

Strauss et al (1997) reported that gastrostomy tube feeding has a negative impact on survival of children with disabilities.[17] They hypothesized that their observed increased mortality risk associated with tube feeding was attributable to respiratory disease secondary to overly vigorous nutritional maintenance and aspiration. This assertion, however, has not been confirmed in other reports that did not find any increase in risk of mortality or respiratory illness in children with cerebral palsy who were fed by gastrostomy.[18]

Clinical observation reveals that some immobile children with spastic quadriplegic cerebral palsy may be overfed via a gastrostomy tube and this accords with research findings. Thus, postoperative follow-up is essential to monitor weight gain (neither too much nor too little) and for the development of 'secondary' GOR . The nursing aspects of gastrostomy feeding are decribed in Chapter 5.

Constipation

Chronic constipation is a common problem in children with disabilities and has been defined as the opening of the bowel less frequently than three times per week or the need for regular laxative treatment. Estimates of the prevalence of constipation vary from 26% to more than 50% for children with severe disabilities.[19]

Contributory factors include prolonged immobility, skeletal abnormalities, extensor spasm or generalized hypotonia, as well as abnormal bowel motility associated with certain neurological lesions.[20] Dietary factors such as low fibre and fluid diets (often because of associated feeding difficulties) are important contributors. The use of anticonvulsant, opioid, antispasmodic, antihistamines or aluminum antacid medications in disabled children may also predispose to constipation.

Constipation in disabled children may be overlooked in the presence of more pressing medical concerns or the inability of the child to communicate effectively. The consequences of constipation may however have a significant impact on the child's well-being. Chronic constipation has been associated with impaired quality of life, urinary symptoms (e.g. poorly voiding bladder, recurrent urinary tract infection and deterioration of vesicoureteric reflux) as well as gastrointestinal manifestations (e.g. recurrent vomiting, chronic nausea, chronic or recurrent abdominal pain and early satiety) .

Assessment of the disabled child with constipation

In addition to a detailed clinical assessment by history and examination, investigations may be useful. Assessment of colonic motility may be performed either with ingestion of radio-opaque markers followed by serial radiographs or by colonic and anorectal manometry. Demonstrated abnormalities of colonic motility associated with neurological impairment include prolongation of colonic transit time in individuals with spinal cord injury or myelomeningocele. The investigation of constipation is described further in Chapter 7.

Treatment of chronic constipation

Treatment of chronic constipation requires a consistent approach and willing parents or carers. Constipation has often gone unrecognized for many months or years in the disabled child and may have resulted in complications such as megarectum, altered bowel motility, anal fissure and soiling. Management of chronic constipation aims to evacuate retained faeces followed by maintenance therapy to ensure defecation is regular and painless. The use of a diary detailing the bowel habit, frequency, size and consistency of stools as well as the laxative treatment used can be helpful to both parents and physicians in assessing the response to treatment.

Initial approach

In children with mild constipation and no evidence of megarectum or soiling the approach is simply to ensure the regular passage of soft stool. Initial attention should be directed towards dietary manipulations. In disabled children who are fed solely via gastrostomy the approach is the usage of a formula with added fibre.

Once dietary issues have been addressed, a stool softener such as lactulose may be used. This synthetic disaccharide is fermented by colonic bacteria and results in an osmotic diarrhoea. The aim is for a porridge-like consistency of stool which is able to be passed without discomfort. Gas is produced as a result of the bacterial fermentation which may result in side effects of abdominal distension and pain. The use of preparations containing polyethylene glycol or paraffin oil should be avoided in children with concomitant neurological abnormalities and gastro-oesophageal reflux due to the significantly increased risk of aspiration.

Stimulant medications may also be required. A mild stimulant such as senna may be helpful in ensuring that defecation occurs at least three times a week. Carers should be informed that colicky abdominal pain may occur with the use of stimulant medications especially in the continued presence of firm stools. If this side effect is seen, attention should be given to softening the stool further and if pain continues, the dose of stimulant may be reduced.

Second-line treatment

In children with rectal impaction and megarectum, disimpaction should firstly be attempted. The use of sodium citrate or sodium acid phosphate enemas is an effective way to clear the rectum before commencing stool softeners and stimulant medication. Enemas may be given under mild sedation if the child is likely to become distressed.

Docusate sodium is a synthetic anionic detergent that decreases surface tension allowing penetration of water and fat into faeces. It is thought to have both stool softening and stimulant properties and may be useful in children who have failed to respond to first-line treatments. Psyllium husk consists of the ground husk of the psyllium seed and is a useful source of soluble fibre.

Soiling results from chronic untreated constipation and is associated with a significant degree of faecal loading. Often local enema treatment is ineffective in treating these patients especially if faecal mass extends throughout the colon.

In patients with an anal fissure, treatment should firstly address their constipation with the use of stool softeners. Topical lignocaine may lessen pain on defecation and topical glycerine trinitrate (GTN) has been used to relax the internal anal sphincter. The use of GTN is limited by the side effect of headache. Injection of botulinum toxin into the anal sphincter is a relatively novel treatment which has been shown in adult studies to be more effective in treating anal fissure than GTN. Botulinum toxin works by blockade of sympathetic (noradrenergic) neural output and therefore may have a role in patients with increased anal sphincter tone because of spinal cord lesions.

SURGICAL TREATMENT

Surgery is usually reserved for patients who have failed medical management especially those with spinal cord lesions. The original Malone antegrade continence enema procedure relied on a reversed appendix brought to the skin to form a stoma. There have been some surgical adaptations since the procedure was originally described and there is now a laparoscopic technique available as well as a percutaneous left colonic approach producing a percutaneous colostomy. A catheter may be introduced through the stoma allowing lavage of saline, phosphate enema solution or polyethylene glycol to achieve defecation. The antegrade continence enema procedure has an 80% reported success rate. Best results are achieved in children more than 5 years old with a neuropathic bowel or anorectal malformation who are highly motivated to remain continent.

References

1. Staiano A, Cucchiara S, Del Giudice E, Andreotti MR, Minella R. Disorders of oesophageal motility in children with psychomotor retardation and gastro-oesophageal reflux. *Eur J Pediatr* 1991; **150**: 638–41.
2. Werlin SL. Antroduodenal motility in neurologically handicapped children with feeding intolerance. *BMC Gastroenterol* 2004; **4**:19.
3. Del Giudice E, Staiano A, Capano G et al. Gastrointestinal manifestations in children with cerebral palsy. *Brain Dev* 1999; **21**: 307–11.
4. Smith CD, Othersen HB, Jr, Gogan N J, Walker JD. Nissen fundoplication in children with profound neurologic disability. High risks and unmet goals. *Ann Surg* 1992; **215**: 654–8.
5. Fonkalsrud EW, Ament ME, Vargas J. Gastric antroplasty for the treatment of delayed gastric emptying and gastro-oesophageal reflux in children. *Am J Surg* 1992; **164**: 327–31.
6. Maxson RT, Harp S, Jackson RJ, Smith SD, Wagner CW. Delayed gastric emptying in neurologically impaired children with gastro-oesophageal reflux: the role of pyloroplasty. *J Pediatr Surg* 1994; **29**: 726–9.
7. Richards CA, Andrews PL, Spitz L, Milla PJ. Nissen fundoplication may induce gastric myoelectrical disturbance in children. *J Pediatr Surg* 1998; **33**: 1801–5.
8. Richards C, Milla P, Andrews P, Spitz, L. Retching and vomiting in neurologically impaired children after fundoplication: Predictive preoperative factors. *J Pediatr Surg* 2001; **36**: 1401–4.
9. Hassall E. Decisions in diagnosing and managing chronic gastro-oesophageal reflux disease in children. *J Pediatr* 2005; **146** (suppl 3): S3–12.
10. Pritchard DS, Baber N, Stephenson T. Should domperidone be used for the treatment of gastro-oesophageal reflux in children? Systematic review of randomized controlled trials in children aged 1 month to 11 years old. *Br J Clin Pharmacol* 2005; **59**: 725–9.
11. Martinez DA, Ginn-Pease, ME, Caniano DA. Sequelae of antireflux surgery in profoundly disabled children. *J Pediatr Surg* 1992; **27**: 267–71.
12. Martinez DA, Ginn-Pease ME, Caniano DA. Recognition of recurrent gastro-oesophageal reflux following antireflux surgery in the neurologically disabled child: high index of suspicion and definitive evaluation. *J Pediatr Surg* 1992; **27**: 983–8.
13. Richards CA, Carr D, Spitz L, Milla PJ, Andrews PL. Nissen-type fundoplication and its effects on the emetic reflex and gastric motility in the ferret. *Neurogastroenterol Motil* 2000; **12**: 1–74.
14. Smith SW, Camfield C, Camfield P. Living with cerebral palsy and tube feeding. A population-based follow-up study. *J Pediatr* 1999; **135**: 307–10.
15. Wheatley MJ, Wesley JR, Tkach DM, Coran AG. Long-term follow-up of brain-damaged children requiring feeding gastrostomy: should an antireflux procedure always be performed? *J Pediatr Surg* 1991; **26**: 301–4.

16. Samson-Fang L, Butler C, O'Donnell M. Effects of gastrostomy feeding in children with cerebral palsy: an AACPDM evidence report. *Dev Med Child Neurol* 2003; **45**: 415–26.

17. Strauss D, Kastner T, Ashwal S, White J. Tubefeeding and mortality in children with severe disabilities and mental retardation. *Pediatrics* 1997; **99**: 358–62.

18. Fung KP, Seagram G, Pasieka J, Trevenen C, Machida H, Scott B. Investigation and outcome of 121 infants and children requiring Nissen fundoplication for the management of gastro-oesophageal reflux. *Clin Invest Med* 1990; **13**: 237–46.

19. Elawad ME, Sullivan PB. Management of constipation in children with disabilities. *Dev Med Child Neurol* 2001; **43**: 829–2.

20. Staiano A, Del Giudice E. Colonic transit and anorectal manometry in children with severe brain damage. *Pediatrics* 1994; **94**: 169–73.

Chapter 7

Gastrointestinal Disorders: Special investigations

Astor Rodrigues

Introduction

It is not surprising that gastrointestinal problems are common in children with neurological impairment given that the enteric nervous system contains more neurons than the spinal cord.[1] In fact, Del Giudice et al's study found that 92% of children with cerebral palsy had clinically significant gastrointestinal symptoms.[2] Gastrointestinal disorders affecting children with neurological impairment include feeding and swallowing difficulties, gastro-oesophageal reflux (GOR) and its complications, abdominal pain and constipation. Needless to say, such difficulties have an impact on their nutritional intake with consequent faltering growth, particularly in the severely disabled children, as has been shown by the Oxford Feeding Study project and other researchers.[3–6] Furthermore, it can also affect the quality of life of the child and their carers.

There is an increased incidence of children with neurological impairment in the general population as a result of a greater number of extremely preterm children surviving their difficult neonatal period.[7] Moreover, with better facilities, these children live longer.[8,9] Unfortunately, sooner or later many of these children run into gastrointestinal difficulties. These difficulties are best assessed by a multidisciplinary feeding team comprising a paediatrician with a special interest in gastroenterology and nutrition, a dietician, a nurse specialist experienced in dealing with tube feeding and a speech and language therapist.

When investigating a child with neurological impairment, a comprehensive history and meticulous clinical examination remain the cornerstone of any assessment. Symptoms and signs of gastrointestinal disorders in these children have been dealt with in some detail in the previous chapter. It is important to remember that although some symptoms evidently point to certain gastrointestinal problem (such as vomiting which may result from GOR or straining and difficulty in passing faeces which may be because of constipation), at other times, especially in those with severe learning difficulties and severe disability, non-specific symptoms such as unsettled behaviour, crying or screaming in pain, food refusal or feeding difficulties bring the child to medical attention and may be representative of certain diagnoses.

Depending on clinical suspicion, appropriate investigations should be undertaken not only to confirm a suspected diagnosis but also to aid management decisions. It is also essential to combine the results of the feeding history, clinical feeding evaluation and results of investigations to arrive at a working diagnosis. It is important for the clinician and the multidisciplinary team requesting investigations to have a sound knowledge of the tests, their advantages and limitations so that the correct test is requested for a suspected condition as well as utilizing the results for effective treatment strategies. Often there are several tests that may provide similar information, hence a clear indication for a particular test and consideration of what question needs to be answered is essential in selecting the appropriate investigation. The specific investigations for gastrointestinal problems in the child with neurological impairment are considered below.

Feeding difficulties

Investigations that may be used to assess feeding problems in children with neurological impairment include a videofluoroscopic swallowing study (VFSS), and pulse oximetry with or without a cardiorespiratory monitor. Polysomnograms may be necessary for obtaining in-depth physiological data, although this is rarely used in clinical practice.

The videofluoroscopic swallowing study (VFSS)

Prior to starting investigations, a clinical evaluation of swallowing preferably by a speech and language therapist is considered useful. This has been discussed in some detail in Chapter 3. A VFSS is essentially undertaken to evaluate the pharyngeal phase of swallowing. The study also helps to document whether pulmonary aspiration is occurring, the reason for it and response to treatment techniques (see Box 7.1).[10,11]

Indications for a VFSS include a history of choking, spluttering or appearing uncomfortable with feeds. VFSS should also be considered in children with more subtle symptoms such as feed refusal, difficulty managing oral secretions and pulmonary complications such as recurrent chest infections, chronic wheezing or breathlessness. In general, in children with neurological impairment there should be a low threshold to request a VFSS especially to determine occult aspiration.

The procedure involves placing the infant or child in a semi-reclined position and obtaining recorded enhanced images during feeding. Swallowing of thicker consistencies should be assessed first (bread or biscuits spread with barium or yogurt mixed with barium) as aspiration is more likely to occur with thin fluids. Thinner liquids mixed with barium/water soluble contrast are then fed using appropriate measures (by spoon or beaker).

Specific observable problems include poor tongue movements, delayed swallow reflex, reduced laryngeal elevation, and silent aspiration.[12] The result of these studies can be of vital importance to the future management of the child, for example, determining the safest position for feeding, which will help prevent long-term aspiration and malnutrition.[10,11] Furthermore, results suggesting an unsafe swallow may aid parental and professional decisions regarding the need for gastrostomy tube feeding.

Pulse oximetry

Pulse oximetry with or without cardiorespiratory monitoring may prove a useful adjunct to the clinical history in determining whether feeding produces physiological changes suggesting swallowing difficulties (see Box 7.2). Furthermore, changes during feeding may also suggest pain from GOR.

The pulse oximeter measures the percentage of oxygen in the capillary blood flow. In normal circumstances, oxygen saturations lie above 95%. After obtaining a baseline reading, feeding is commenced and monitoring is continued. Changes such as

Box 7.1 Advantages and disadvantages of VFSS

Advantages:

- provides a detailed assessment of the pharyngeal swallow with different food consistencies, textures and feeding positions;
- effectiveness of treatment techniques can be observed during the study.

Disadvantages/limitations:

- the viscosity of barium may alter the child's swallowing response and may appear normal although difficulties are recognized clinically;
- the relatively brief period of the study may not be a true representation of the actual problems;
- it does not identify structural abnormalities of the pharynx or oesophagus.

Box 7.2 Advantages and disadvantages of pulse oximetry

Advantages:

- non-invasive and portable;
- can help determine the significance of problems coordinating swallowing;
- more reliable than observing colour change.

Disadvantages/limitations:

- affected by movement and perfusion;
- does not identify the nature of the pathology causing the physiological changes.

desaturations, bradycardia and increased respiratory effort during feeding may suggest swallowing difficulties.

Gastro-oesophageal reflux disease

Gastro-oesophageal reflux disease (GORD) is common in children with neurological impairment and various studies in children with cerebral palsy suggest a high prevalence.[13,14] Several causes of GORD in this group of children have been suggested. These include impairment of both lower oesophageal sphincter function and oesophageal peristalsis, increased intra-abdominal pressure secondary to spasticity and scoliosis, prolonged adoption of the supine position and seizure. The effective management of GOR in children with neurological impairment is vital as this group is at higher risk of severe GORD and its resultant complications. GORD even in neurological impairment children may be occult and present with non-specific symptoms such as chronic irritability, unexplained crying, food refusal, and apparent dystonic movements (Sandifer's syndrome). Therefore, a high index of suspicion should be maintained when assessing these children to diagnose GOR.

The various symptoms of GOR are detailed in Box 7.3.

Box 7.3 Symptoms of gastro-oesophageal reflux

1. Oesophageal symptoms:
   Specific symptoms:
   - nausea, vomiting, regurgitation.

   Non-specific symptoms possibly related to oesophagitis:
   - dysphagia;
   - epigastric, retrosternal pain/chest pain (heartburn);
   - iron deficiency anaemia;
   - haematemesis, melena;
   - weight loss, faltering growth;
   - feeding difficulties/food refusal.
2. Extra-oesophageal symptoms:
   - wheezing, recurrent pneumonia;
   - aspiration pneumonia;
   - otitis media;
   - chronic sinusitis;
   - laryngitis;
   - laryngomalacia;
   - subglottic oedema and stenosis;
   - dental erosions.

The following investigations should be considered in a child with neurological impairment to establish the diagnosis of GORD.

Twenty-four-hour lower oesophageal pH monitoring

This test is widely available and still remains one of the best tests to demonstrate the presence of acid in the lower oesophagus which correlates well with acid reflux. The indications for a 24-hour pH study in children with neurological impairment include establishing whether non-specific symptoms such as unexplained crying, unsettled behaviour, dystonic posturing etc. are a result of GOR. Additionally, it may also be useful prior to a gastrostomy insertion and if significant reflux is detected, a fundoplication may be required as well.

PRE-PROCEDURE PREPARATION

Except for fasting for at least 3 to 5 hours before the study to avoid nausea and vomiting, no other special preparation is necessary for pH monitoring. In children capable of communication, it is important to explain the procedure and reassure the child at the beginning of the study. It may be distressing for a parent or caregiver to witness the pH probe insertion and a prior explanation may prove useful to dispel any anxieties. The child and family should be forewarned that the passage of the pH probe through the throat is uncomfortable at first, although after a few minutes, they would get accustomed to it. To facilitate insertion, a lubricant water-soluble jelly or silicone spray can be placed on the electrode, avoiding the pH sensor. A sedative is not advisable as it may interfere with swallowing and influence lower oesophageal pressures resulting in an unreliable result. Antacids are allowed up to 6 hours prior to the start of the recording. H-2 (Histamine-2) receptor blockers or proton pump inhibitors (PPIs) should be stopped at least 3 or 7 days respectively, prior to the procedure. Prokinetics should be stopped at least 48 hours before the pH monitoring. Ideally, a pH study should be avoided on the same day as an upper gastrointestinal endoscopy as sedation or anaesthesia and inflated air may influence the results.

PH PROBE LOCATION

Oesophageal location of the electrode is of vital importance and influences the number and duration of acid reflux episodes recorded. The proximity of the electrode to the lower oesophageal sphincter directly influences the number of acid reflux episodes recorded. In children fluoroscopy, manometry, endoscopy and calculation of the oesophageal length according to the Strobel's formula – distance from the nose to the cardia = 5 + [0.252 × (height (cms)] – are among several methods that have been proposed to establish the location of the pH probe. Manometry in infants and children is time consuming, invasive, inherently difficult to obtain and most importantly, would not be suited to locate the ideal position of the probe (from a fixed point) because of the variable lengths of children's oesophagus. Endoscopy on the other hand has its own risks and may involve sedation or general anaesthesia. Therefore, fluoroscopy which involves minimal radiation has been recommended by the European Society for Paediatric Gastroenterology, Hepatology, and Nutrition Working Group on GOR to determine the final position of the probe. The tip should be situated in such a way that it overlies the third vertebral body above the diaphragm both during inspiration and expiration.

PROCEDURE

The pH recording device and the pH probe are calibrated using standardized pH solutions. Once the probe position is confirmed the recording is begun. The duration of the recording should include a day and a night period and be at least 18 hours if a 24 hour recording is not possible. No special changes in the child's diet or position are necessary and the family should be encouraged to keep to the usual routine. Hot and cold beverages should be avoided as they could damage the probe. Hospitalization is not required in most cases and in our centre parents are encouraged to continue the recording at home. After the recording, the data are downloaded on to a computer using a special program for analysis (Figure 7.1).

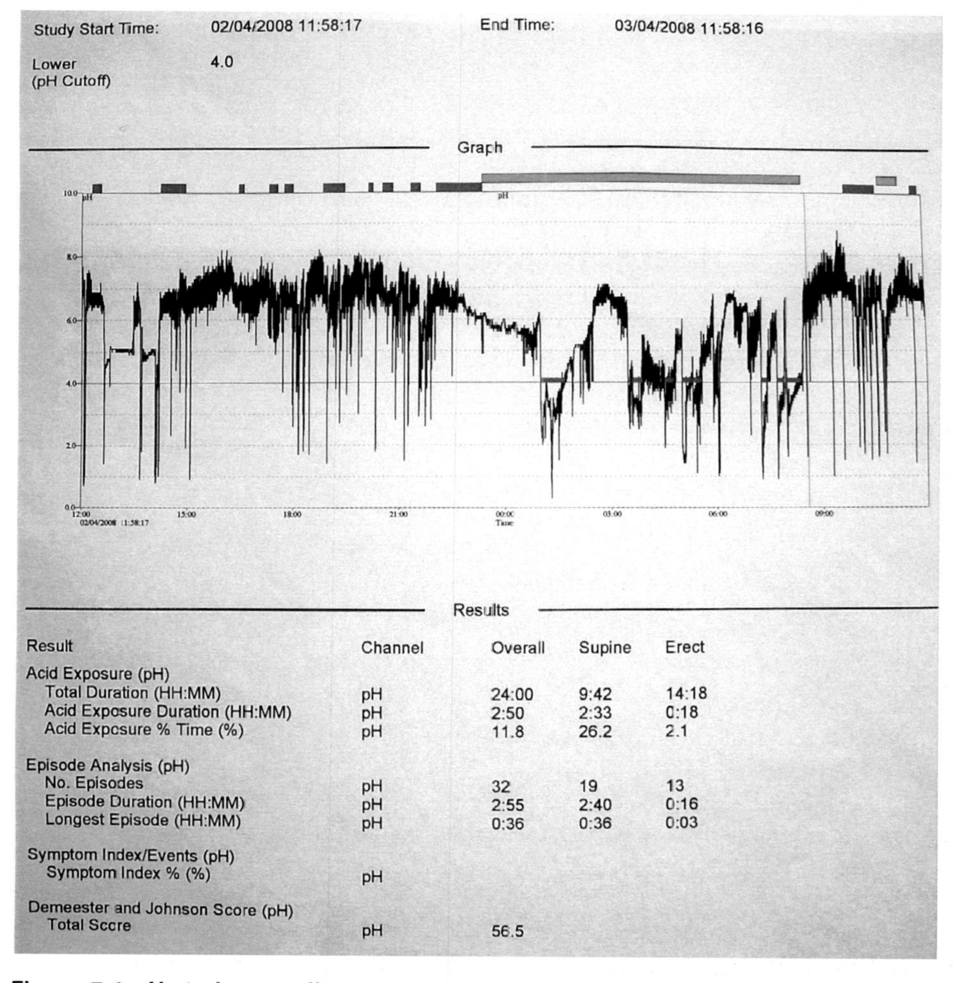

Study Start Time: 02/04/2008 11:58:17 End Time: 03/04/2008 11:58:16

Lower (pH Cutoff) 4.0

Graph

Results

Result	Channel	Overall	Supine	Erect
Acid Exposure (pH)				
Total Duration (HH:MM)	pH	24:00	9:42	14:18
Acid Exposure Duration (HH:MM)	pH	2:50	2:33	0:18
Acid Exposure % Time (%)	pH	11.8	26.2	2.1
Episode Analysis (pH)				
No. Episodes	pH	32	19	13
Episode Duration (HH:MM)	pH	2:55	2:40	0:16
Longest Episode (HH:MM)	pH	0:36	0:36	0:03
Symptom Index/Events (pH)				
Symptom Index % (%)	pH			
Demeester and Johnson Score (pH)				
Total Score	pH	56.5		

Figure 7.1 pH study recording.

DATA ANALYSIS

The parameters that are typically analysed are:

- total number of reflux episodes,
- number of reflux episodes lasting more than 5 minutes,
- duration of the longest reflux episode;
- reflux index (percentage of time of the entire duration of the investigation during which the pH is less than 4.0).

The reflux index is perhaps the most useful and indicative of the severity of GOR.

In general, it can be stated that a reflux index above 10% should be considered as abnormal, a reflux index below 5% as normal.[15] Studies in children with neurological impairment demonstrated that the majority of reflux episodes are non-acidic and are missed using conventional pH monitoring (see Box 7.4).[16]

Multichannel intraluminal impedance study

The method is based on measuring the resistance to alternating current (i.e. impedance) of the content of the oesophageal lumen by detecting intraoesophageal bolus (solid, liquid, gas) movement. Multichannel intraluminal impedance can be added to conventional pH catheters, allowing a more comprehensive characterization of reflux episodes, including physical properties (i.e. liquid, gas, mixed), chemical properties (i.e. acid or non-acid), height of the refluxate, bolus presence and clearance, and acid presence and clearance. Del Buono and colleagues looking at impedance studies in children with neurological impairment concluded that more than half of the reflux

Box 7.4 Advantages and disadvantages of 24-hour pH monitoring

Advantages:

- it helps to confirm and quantify acid reflux;
- it may suggest oesophageal dysmotility if prolonged reflux episodes are detected;
- the relationship of reflux episodes to symptoms (pain, posturing, apnoeas, etc.) could be determined;
- it may help to decide on the need for a fundoplication, if a gastrostomy is needed.

Disadvantages/limitations:

- it may be technically difficult to perform in children with spinal deformities;
- it does not demonstrate non-acid reflux;
- it does not measure the volume or distance covered by the refluxate;
- it cannot detect complications of GORD (e.g. oesophagitis).

events were non-acidic and would therefore go undetected by conventional pH study.[16] There were more reflux events in children fed nasogastrically than oral-fed children. Published data using this technique are still limited in children with neurological impairment and whether it will prove superior to a pH study to aid clinical decisions is yet to be seen.

Upper gastrointestinal endoscopy with biopsy

Endoscopy, particularly when supplemented by histology, is the most precise method of indicating oesophageal damage by reflux.[17] Direct visualization of the oesophageal mucosa can assess the presence and severity of oesophagitis, strictures and Barrett's oesophagus. It is, however, important to remember that these children may have underlying lung/airway disease from chronic aspiration with poor respiratory reserve and poor cardiac reserve from malnutrition making sedation/general anaesthesia more risky (see Box 7.5).

Microscopic evaluation of biopsy samples from the distal oesophagus demonstrates abnormalities in many children with neurological impairment who have symptoms but no endoscopically visualized erosions. Infiltration of the epithelium with inflammatory cells, such as neutrophils and eosinophils, not normally present in the epithelium of young children, can be used as indicators of GORD. Intraepithelial lymphocytes are more sensitive than other inflammatory cells but are fairly common; their specificity for GORD remains unclear. Morphometric histological parameters require adequate size and proper orientation of the biopsy specimens but seem more reliable for the diagnosis of GORD.[18]

Upper gastrointestinal contrast study

Also known as a barium/contrast meal, this test is specific but not sensitive enough to diagnose GOR (see Box 7.6).[19] It involves swallowing a radio-opaque contrast substance

Box 7.5 Advantages and disadvantages of upper gastrointestinal endoscopy with biopsy

Advantages:

- macroscopic and microscopic assessment of the oesophagus can better define the severity and extent of GORD;
- effect of treatment may be studied objectively on repeat endoscopy.

Disadvantages/limitations:

- invasive;
- needs anaesthesia/sedation with accompanying risks;
- inter-observer variation in macroscopic and histological interpretations.

Box 7.6 Advantages and disadvantages of an upper gastrointestinal contrast study

Advantages:
- useful investigation if a cause other than GOR is suspected;
- useful before anti-reflux surgery to exclude anomalies of the upper gastrointestinal tract such as malrotation, duodenal stenosis and hiatus hernia.

Disadvantages/limitations:
- exposure to radiation greater than other tests;
- not sensitive for GOR.

to outline the anatomy of the upper gastrointestinal tract. In children with neurological impairment with concerns of an unsafe swallow, the contrast may be instilled through a nasogastric tube. This may, however, preclude visualization of the oesophageal phase of swallowing and may not prove useful to study conditions affecting the oesophagus such as strictures, achalasia, vascular rings and oesophageal dysmotility.

Scintigraphy for gastro-oesophageal reflux
This test is also known as the 'milk scan' as milk is often used as the feed to which the radioisotope is mixed. For GOR scintigraphy, oral technetium-99m sulfur colloid or phytate colloids mixed with feeds are used because they are not absorbed from the gastrointestinal tract. Moreover, if aspirated, they are readily demonstrable, and are ultimately cleared without consequence. After the labelled colloid is mixed with the feed to be administered, it is introduced in the stomach orally or via a nasogastric or gastrostomy feeding tube. Any remaining activity is cleared from the mouth and oesophagus with an unlabelled liquid or feed, and the patient is imaged for 1 hour using a gamma camera.

Dynamic images are then obtained at regular intervals, usually over a 1-hour period. Both images and time-activity curves are recorded, which enables the identification of the frequency of reflux episodes together with their proximal extent.

Using this method, the results obtained can be considered to represent only the postprandial situation. Although, pulmonary aspiration may occasionally be detected on delayed images of the thorax (1 and 4 hours after the study), the sensitivity of this as a diagnostic test is poor (see Box 7.7).

SCINTIGRAPHY FOR GASTRIC EMPTYING
Scintigraphic assessment of gastric emptying in association with the evaluation of GOR is also feasible, but its value must be considered questionable. Gastric emptying studies may be useful in selected patients, for example, when considering gastrostomy

Box 7.7 Advantages and disadvantages of scintigraphy

Advantages:

- useful to detect reflux in the postprandial period when the pH of the stomach is neutralized by food and pH study may not detect reflux (i.e. detects both acid and alkaline reflux);
- able to measure the height of the refluxate;
- radiation exposure considerably less that barium studies;
- delayed images may reveal evidence of pulmonary aspiration.

Disadvantages/limitations:

- the period of the study may not be sufficient to demonstrate GOR, which is by nature intermittent;
- does not detect anatomical abnormalities such as hiatus hernia, malrotation etc.;
- does not provide information regarding the length of the reflux episode;
- false positive rates may be high, as children are laid in the supine position under the gamma camera, which may exacerbate reflux.

placement, when considering fundoplication and evaluating patients with dumping syndrome.[20] The procedure is similar to that used for studying GOR as described above. If gastric emptying is roughly 50% at 1 hour, the study can be terminated. If there is delayed emptying at 1 hour, the patient is allowed to sit upright or walk around before delayed images are acquired at 90 minutes and 2 hours.

Children with delayed gastric emptying may be at a greater risk of developing retching and gas-bloat syndrome after fundoplication. If delayed gastric emptying has been demonstrated, consideration should be given to whether or not to perform a pyloroplasty. Evidence for the effectiveness of this approach, however, is at present controversial.[21,22]

Oesophageal manometry and ultrasound scans have also been used to diagnose GOR, however this is not common practice.

In fact, a study comparing the accuracy of diagnostic tests (prior to the advent of multichannel impedance study) in infants and children with GOR concluded that the pH study was the most reliable test and correlated best with symptoms of GOR.[23]

Pulmonary involvement from gastrointestinal causes

Children with neurological impairment commonly present with frequent respiratory infections.[24] GOR and aspiration secondary to an unsafe swallow are among several factors contributing to this problem. In children who are exclusively gastrostomy fed, aspiration of saliva may also lead to recurrent chest infections. It is important to ascertain the cause of aspiration, i.e. whether from GOR or swallowing difficulties as the management varies significantly. The following investigations may be considered to determine whether pulmonary disease is linked to problems related to gastrointestinal difficulties.

Bronchoscopy and broncho-alveolar lavage

In children with persisting respiratory problems suspected to be related to GOR, a bronchoscopy may reveal inflammation of the laryngeal inlet and larynx. Examination of fluid produced by broncho-alveolar lavage may reveal presence of fat laden macrophages which suggests pulmonary aspiration. This test, however, does not indicate whether pulmonary aspiration is a result of aspiration during oral feeds or from aspiration of the refluxate. Although this test is not sensitive, a positive result helps confirm pulmonary aspiration.

Scintigraphy for suspected pulmonary aspiration

Delayed images obtained on a 'milk scan' may demonstrate pulmonary aspiration from GOR, albeit with a low sensitivity.[25] If there is no strong evidence of GOR clinically or on investigation, a salivagram may be considered. In this test a small amount of labelled colloid is placed on the tongue and is allowed to mix with saliva. Subsequent images of the tracheobronchial tree collected up to an hour afterward may indicate aspiration of saliva. However, the accuracy of this method has not been assessed.

Constipation

Up to three-quarters of children with cerebral palsy are chronically constipated.[2] Predisposing factors are multiple and include:

- nutritional factors, for example diet, including proprietary enteral feeds, that are low in fibre, poor fluid intake;
- pharmacological factors, for example anticholinergics, opiates, baclofen, valproic acid;
- mobility factors, inability to sit/squat on the toilet eliminating the effects of gravity and stability of the rectum); and
- neuromuscular factors, for example hypotonia, skeletal muscle incoordination, skeletal deformities and neuropathic bowel from spinal dysraphism.

Unfortunately, there is often a delay in the recognition and treatment of this problem and symptoms may be present for several months to years. This delay may be as a result of the inability of the child to communicate effectively, or because constipation is accepted as an inevitable consequence of cerebral palsy, or because a higher priority is given to other aspects of their management. Whatever the cause, unnoticed, constipation may result in considerable – and avoidable – distress to the child.

Complications of chronic constipation may result in other gastrointestinal manifestations: chronic nausea, anorexia, recurrent vomiting, chronic or recurrent abdominal pain, and overflow 'spurious' diarrhoea. In addition, urinary difficulties such as recurrent urinary tract infections, incomplete voiding and worsening vesicoureteric reflux may complicate constipation.[26]

Investigations of constipation in children with neurological impairment

On initial assessment, a detailed history is essential. Details of stool frequency, consistency and soiling should be obtained. Any history of delayed passage of meconium (>24 hours after birth) should lead to consideration of a rectal biopsy to rule out Hirschsprung disease. Examination should include a detailed general examination especially for evidence of pallor (consider coeliac disease, lead poisoning) and thyroid swelling (consider hypothyroidism). The presence of hard stools palpable through the abdomen suggests impaction. The presence of fissures or skin tags on perianal examination may provide a clue not only to the aetiology of the constipation but also to the reason for persistence of symptoms or for the active withholding of stools. A patulous anus may indicate underlying neuromuscular pathology in a child with constipation. Digital examination of the rectum may, when hard stools are felt near the anal verge, indicate faecal impaction or suggest anal stenosis or Hirschsprung disease. A thorough clinical history and examination should suffice to make a clear diagnosis of constipation and investigations are not usually necessary. Investigations may be justified, however, in some difficult to examine children.

ABDOMINAL X-RAY

This is useful in assessing the degree of faecal loading especially in children where clinical examination is difficult. It may help influence the choice of treatment as well as indicating to the parents the nature of the problem, especially in those presenting with chronic diarrhoea. Scoring systems to assess faecal loading have been developed and may assist with management strategies.[27,28] Occult spinal anomalies providing clues to spinal dysraphism may also be detected on an abdominal X-ray. The main disadvantage is with the not insignificant exposure to ionizing radiation that is required.

COLONIC TRANSIT TIMES

This can be measured by detecting radio-opaque markers that have been swallowed on days 1, 2 and 3 on an abdominal X-ray obtained at day 5.[29] Delayed proximal colonic transit is frequently observed in children with cerebral palsy and is related to their degree of immobility.[30] Prolonged colonic transit times are also seen in individuals with spinal injury or myelomeningocoele.[31] In children with delayed total or proximal colonic times prokinetic or stimulant laxative therapy should be considered. Surgical intervention (e.g.colostomy) is reserved for the most intractable constipation.

Anorectal manometry

Although not routinely used studies have looked at the anorectal function of children with neurological problems.[31,32] Agnarsson et al (1993) demonstrated a low resting pressure in the first centimetre of the anal canal in children with cerebral palsy with slow anal rhythmical activity; pressure increase in the first centimetre occurred only during maximum rectal distension. These findings suggest anal sphincter and/or pelvic floor muscle incoordination, but no evidence of abnormal rectal function.[32] However, others have found no differences in anal pressures and in the anorectal motor responses to rectal distension in children with neurological impairment and those without, with or without functional constipation.[33]

Conclusion

In summary, engagement of the patient with the multidisciplinary team from the outset is the best model of service. It is essential to acquire a comprehensive history and carry out a meticulous clinical examination to formulate a clear impression of the patient and to arrive at a correct diagnosis. Investigations may help to resolve differential diagnoses and aid management decisions. Their results, however, must be interpreted in the context of the clinical assessment including information provided by the feeding history and clinical feeding evaluation. It is vital for the clinician and the multidisciplinary team to have a firm understanding of the indications for, and advantages and limitations of investigations that they wish to undertake. Similarly, they must have a detailed understanding of the range and effectiveness of treatment strategies.

References

1. Menkes JH, Ament ME. Neurologic disorders of gastroesophageal function. *Adv Neurol* 1988; **49**: 409–16.
2. Del Giudice E, Staiano A, Capano G et al. Gastrointestinal manifestations in children with cerebral palsy. *Brain Dev* 1999; **21**: 307–11.
3. Sullivan PB, Lambert B, Rose M, Ford-Adams M, Johnson A, Griffiths P. Prevalence and severity of feeding and nutritional problems in children with neurological impairment: Oxford Feeding Study. *Dev Med Child Neurol* 2000; **42**: 10–80.
4. Sullivan PB, Juszczak E, Lambert BR, Rose M, Ford-Adams ME, Johnson A. Impact of feeding problems on nutritional intake and growth: Oxford Feeding Study II. *Dev Med Child Neurol* 2002; **44**: 461–7.
5. Thommessen M, Kase BF, Riis G, Heiberg A. The impact of feeding problems on growth and energy intake in children with cerebral palsy. *Eur J Clin Nutr* 1991; **45**: 479–87.
6. Samson-Fang LJ, Stevenson RD. Identification of malnutrition in children with cerebral palsy: poor performance of weight-for-height centiles. *Dev Med Child Neurol* 2000; **42**: 162–8.
7. Tin W, Wariyar U, Hey E. Changing prognosis for babies of less than 28 weeks' gestation in the north of England between 1983 and 1994. *BMJ* 1997; **314**: 107–11.
8. Crichton JU, Mackinnon M, White CP. The life-expectancy of persons with cerebral palsy. *Dev Med Child Neurol* 1995; **37**: 567–76.
9. Hutton JL, Cooke T, Pharoah POD. Life expectancy in children with cerebral palsy. *BMJ* 1994; **309**: 431–5.

10. Wright RE, Wright FR, Carson CA. Videofluoroscopic assessment in children with severe cerebral palsy presenting with dysphagia. *Pediatr Radiol* 1996; **26**: 10–2.

11. Morton RE, Bonas R, Fourie B, Minford J. Videofluoroscopy in the assessment of feeding disorders of children with neurological problems. *Dev Med Child Neurol* 1993; **35**: 388–95.

12. Arvedson J, Lefton-Grief M. *Pediatric videoflu'oscopic swallow studies: A professional manual with caregivers guidelines*. San Antonio, TX: Communication Skill Builders, 1998.

13. Sondheimer JM, Morris BA. Gastroesophageal reflux among severely retarded children. *J Pediatr* 1979; **94**: 710–4.

14. Schwarz SM, Corredor J, Fisher-Medina J, Cohen J, Rabinowitz S. Diagnosis and treatment of feeding disorders in children with developmental disabilities. *Pediatrics* 2001; **108**: 671–6.

15. Sullivan PB. Gastrostomy feeding in the disabled child: when is an antireflux procedure required? *Arch Dis Child* 1999; **81**: 463–4.

16. Del Buono R, Wenzl TG, Rawat D, Thomson M. Acid and nonacid gastro-oesophageal reflux in neurologically impaired children: investigation with the multiple intraluminal impedance procedure. *J Pediatr Gastroenterol Nutr* 2006; **43**: 331–5.

17. Bohmer CJM, Niezen-de Boer MC, Klinkenberg-Knol EC, Deville WLJM, Nadorp JHSM, Meuwissen SGM. The prevalence of gastroesophageal reflux disease in institutionalized intellectually disabled individuals. *Amer J Gastroenterol* 1999; **94**: 804–10.

18. Vandenplas Y, Ashkenazi A, Belli D. A proposition for the diagnosis and treatment of gastro oesophageal disease. Working Group of the European Society of Pediatric Gastro-enterology and Nutrition (ESPGAN). *Eur J Pediatr* 1993; **152**: 704–11.

19. Meyers WF, Roberts CC, Johnson DG, Herbst JJ. Values of tests for evaluation of gastro-esophageal reflux in children. *J Pediatr Surg* 1985; **20**: 515–20.

20. Fonkalsrud EW, Foglia RP, Ament ME, Berquist W, Vargas J. Operative treatment for the gastroesophageal reflux syndrome in children. *J Pediatr Surg* 1989; **24**: 525–9.

21. Fonkalsrud EW, Ament ME, Vargas J. Gastric antroplasty for the treatment of delayed gastric emptying and gastroesophageal reflux in children. *Am J Surg* 1992; **164**: 327–31.

22. Maxson RT, Harp S, Jackson RJ, Smith SD, Wagner CW. Delayed gastric emptying in neurologically impaired children with gastroesophageal reflux: the role of pyloroplasty. *J Pediatr Surg* 1994; **29**: 726–9.

23. Arasu TS, Wyllie R, Fitzgerald JF et al. Gastroesophageal reflux in infants and children comparative accuracy of diagnostic methods. *J Pediatr* 1980; **96**: 798–803.

24. Morton RE, Wheatley R, Minford J. Respiratory tract infections due to direct and reflux aspiration in children with severe neurodisability. *Dev Med Child Neurol* 1999; **41**: 329–34.

25. Ravelli AM, Panarotto MB, Verdoni L, Consolati V, Bolognini S. Pulmonary aspiration shown by scintigraphy in gastroesophageal reflux-related respiratory disease. *Chest* 2006; **130**: 1520–6.

26. Loening-Baucke V. Urinary incontinence and urinary tract infection and their resolution with treatment of chronic constipation of childhood [see comments]. *Pediatrics* 1997; **100**: 228–32.

27. Leech SC, McHugh K, Sullivan PB. Evaluation of a method of assessing faecal loading on plain abdominal radiographs in children. *Pediatr Radiol* 1999; **29**: 255–8.

28. van den BM, Graafmans D, Nievelstein R, Beek E. Systematic assessment of constipation on plain abdominal radiographs in children. *Pediatr Radiol* 2006; **36**: 224–6.

29. Papadopoulou A, Clayden GS, Booth IW. The clinical value of solid marker transit studies in childhood constipation and soiling. *Eur J Pediatr* 1994; **153**: 560–4.

30. Park ES, Park CI, Cho SR, Na SI, Cho YS. Colonic transit time and constipation in children with spastic cerebral palsy. *Arch Phys Med Rehabil* 2004; **85**: 453–6.

31. Agnarsson U, Warde C, McCarthy G, Clayden GS, Evans N. Anorectal function of children with neurological problems. I: Spina bifida. *Dev Med Child Neurol* 1993; **35**: 893–902.

32. Agnarsson U, Warde C, McCarthy G, Clayden GS, Evans N. Anorectal function of children with neurological problems. II: cerebral palsy. *Dev Med Child Neurol* 1993; **35**: 903–8.

33. Staiano A, Del Giudice E. Colonic transit and anorectal manometry in children with severe brain damage. *Pediatrics* 1994; **94**: 169–73.

Appendices

Appendix 1: Cerebral palsy growth charts. Reproduced with permission. Day SM, Strauss DJ, Vachon PJ, Rosenbloom L, Shavelle RM, Wu YW. Growth patterns in a population of children and adolescents with cerebral palsy. *Dev Med Child Neurol* 2007; **49**: 167–171. The full set of charts are also available in PDF at the Life Expectancy Project website: www.LifeExpectancy.org/articles/GrowthCharts.shtml.

Appendix 1: Cerebral palsy growth charts

Appendix 1 i

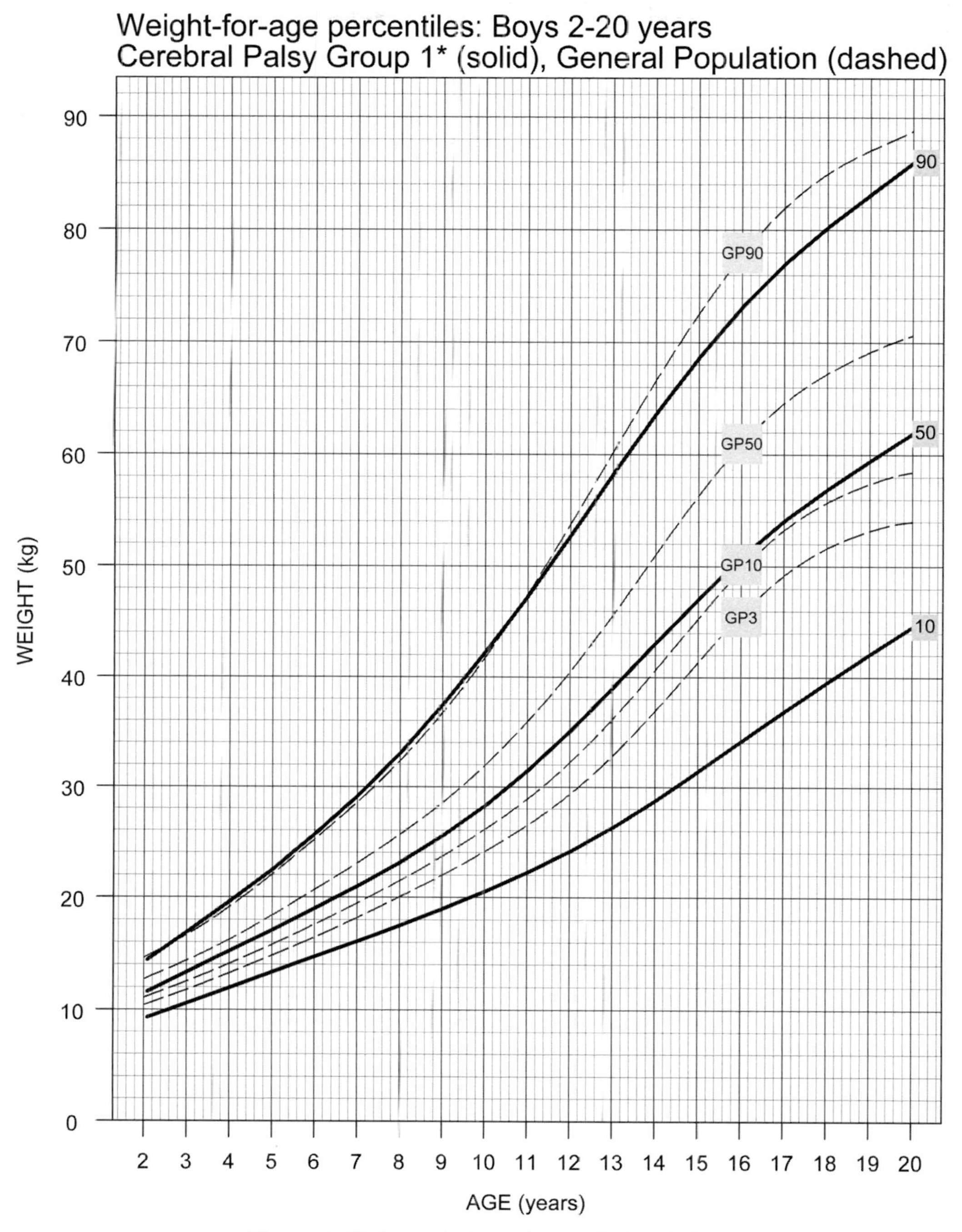

Appendix 1 ii

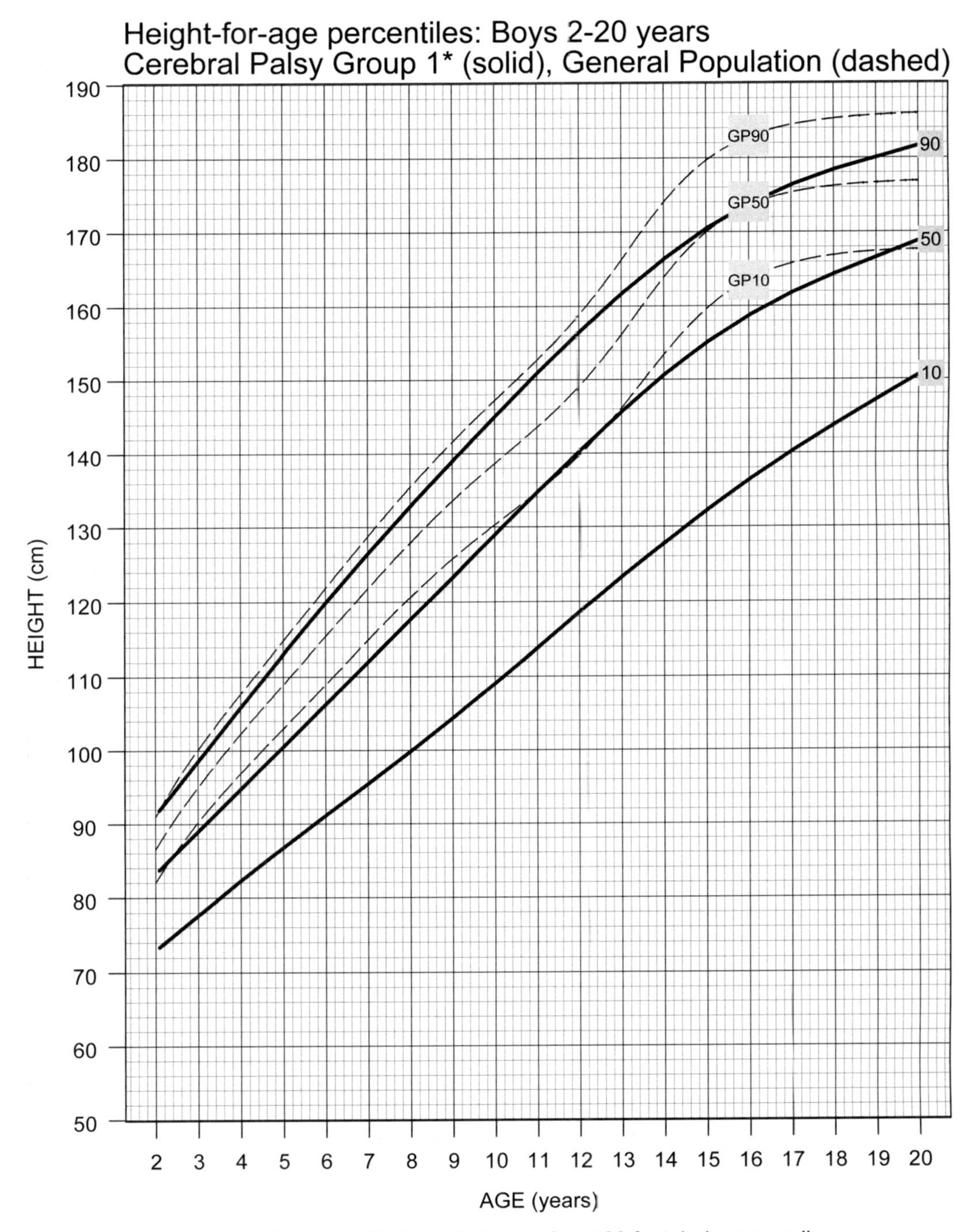

*Group 1: Walks well alone at least 20 feet, balances well.

Appendix 1 iii

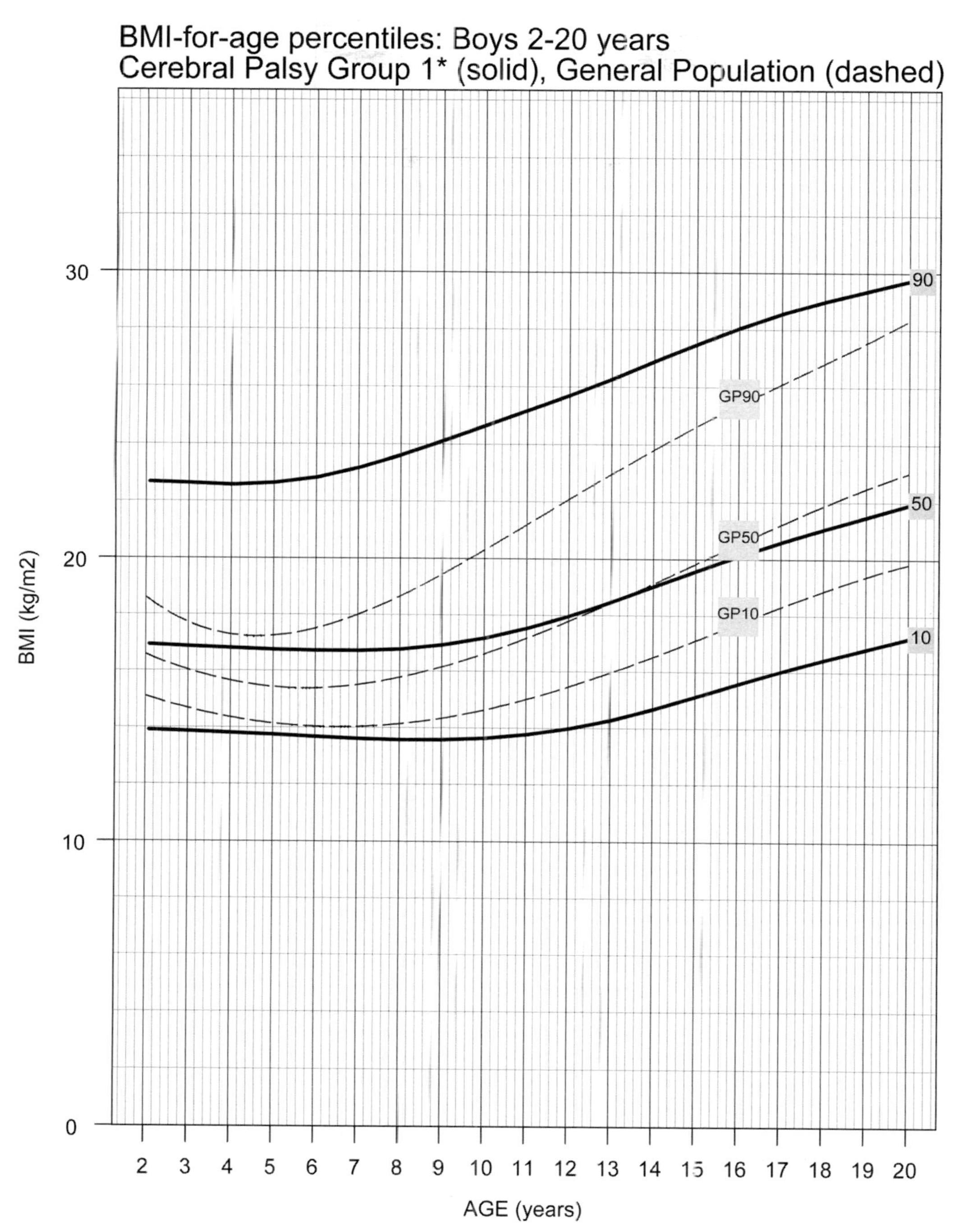

Appendix 1 iv

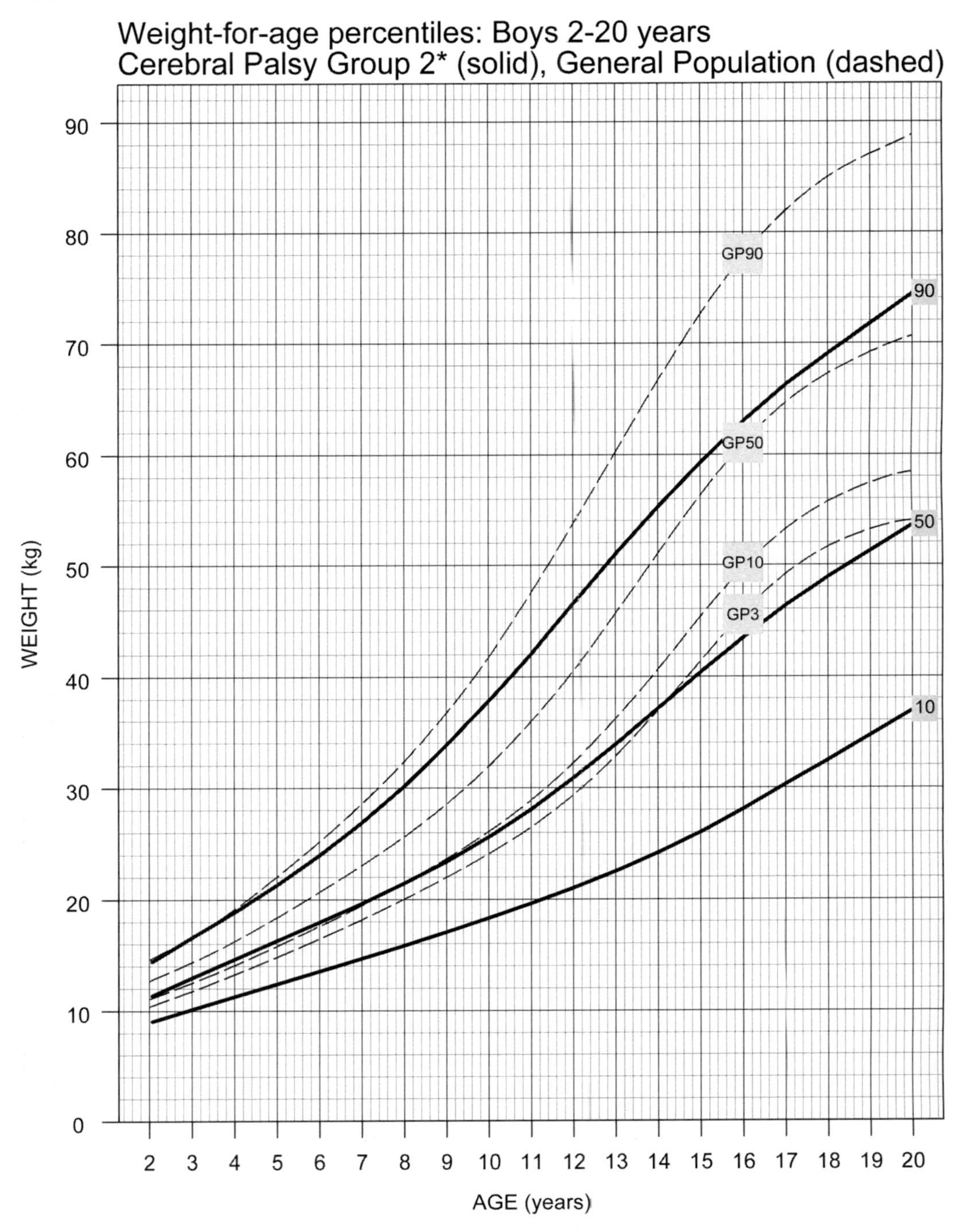

*Group 2: Walks with support or unsteadily alone at least 10 feet.

Appendix 1 v

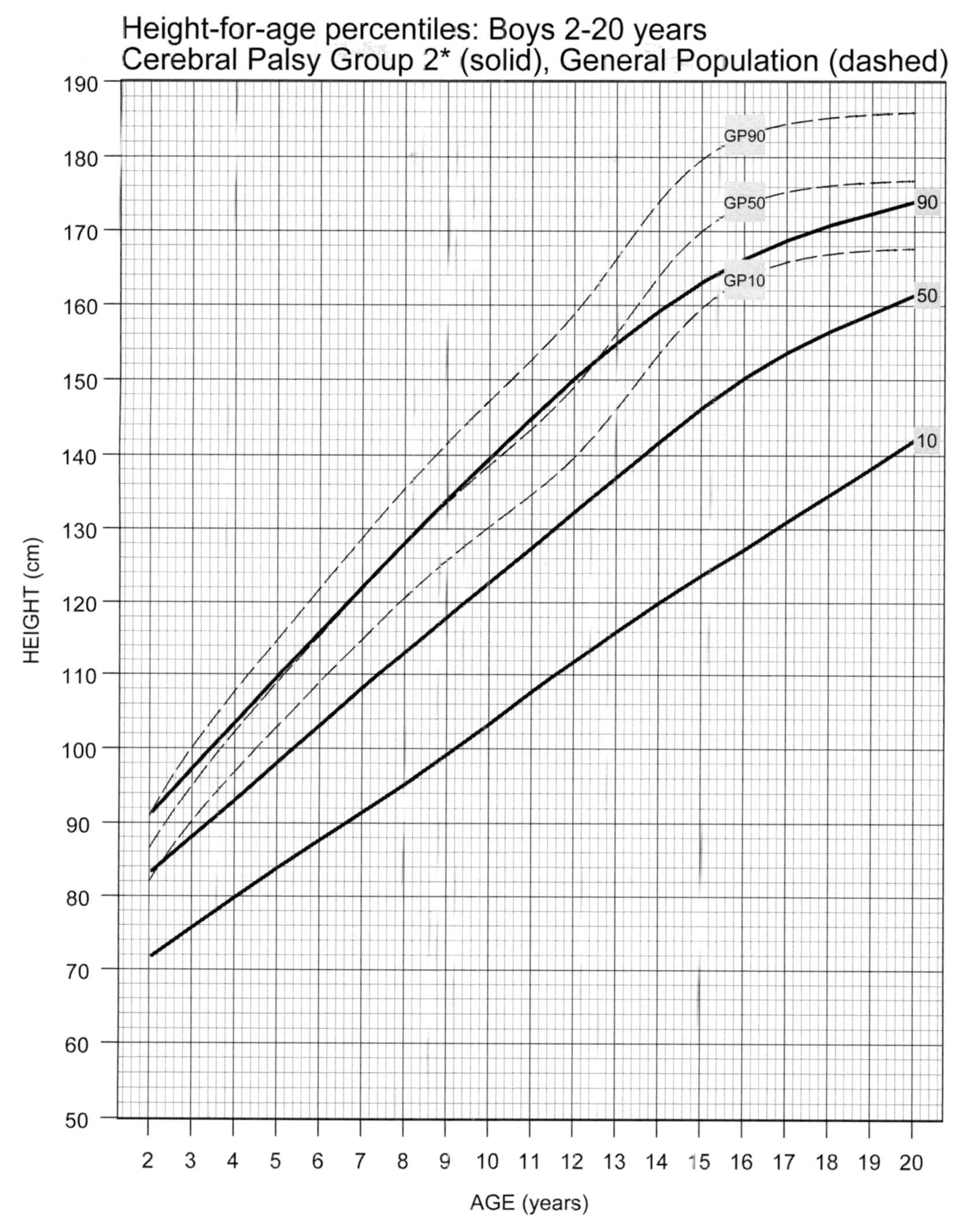

*Group 2: Walks with support or unsteadily alone at least 10 feet.

Appendix 1 vi

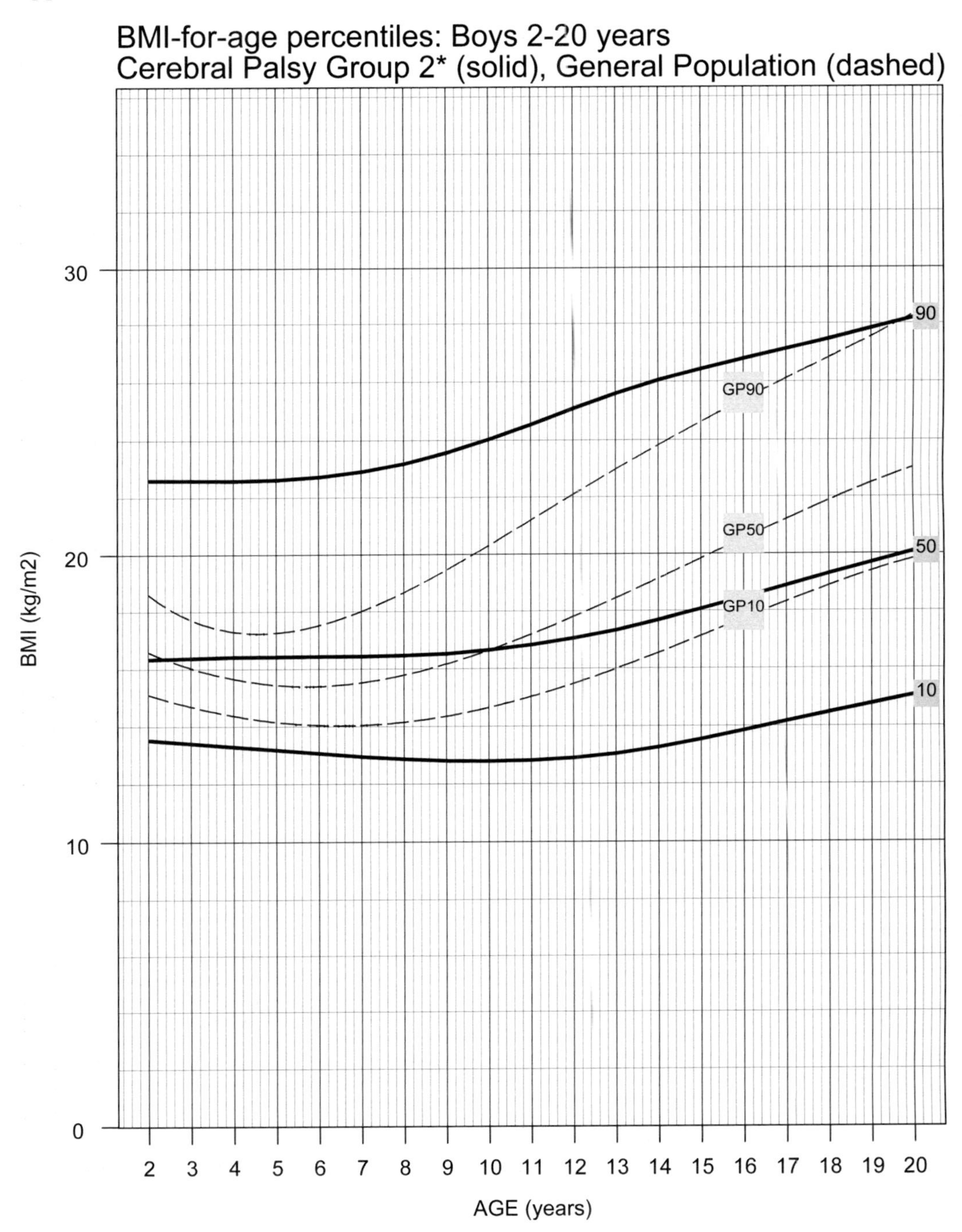

*Group 2: Walks with support or unsteadily alone at least 10 feet.

Appendix 1 vii

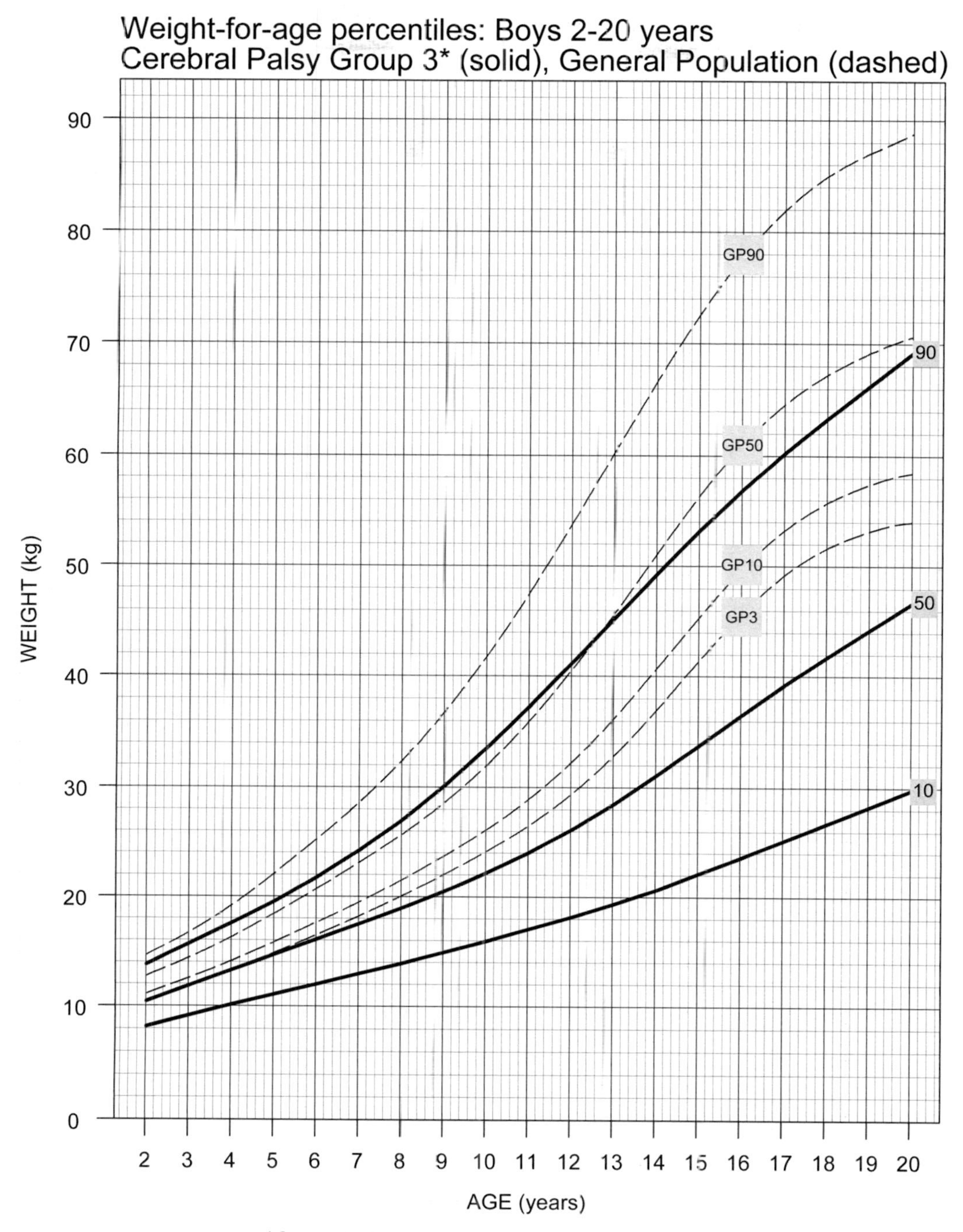

*Group 3: Crawls, creeps or scoots, but does not walk.

Appendix 1 viii

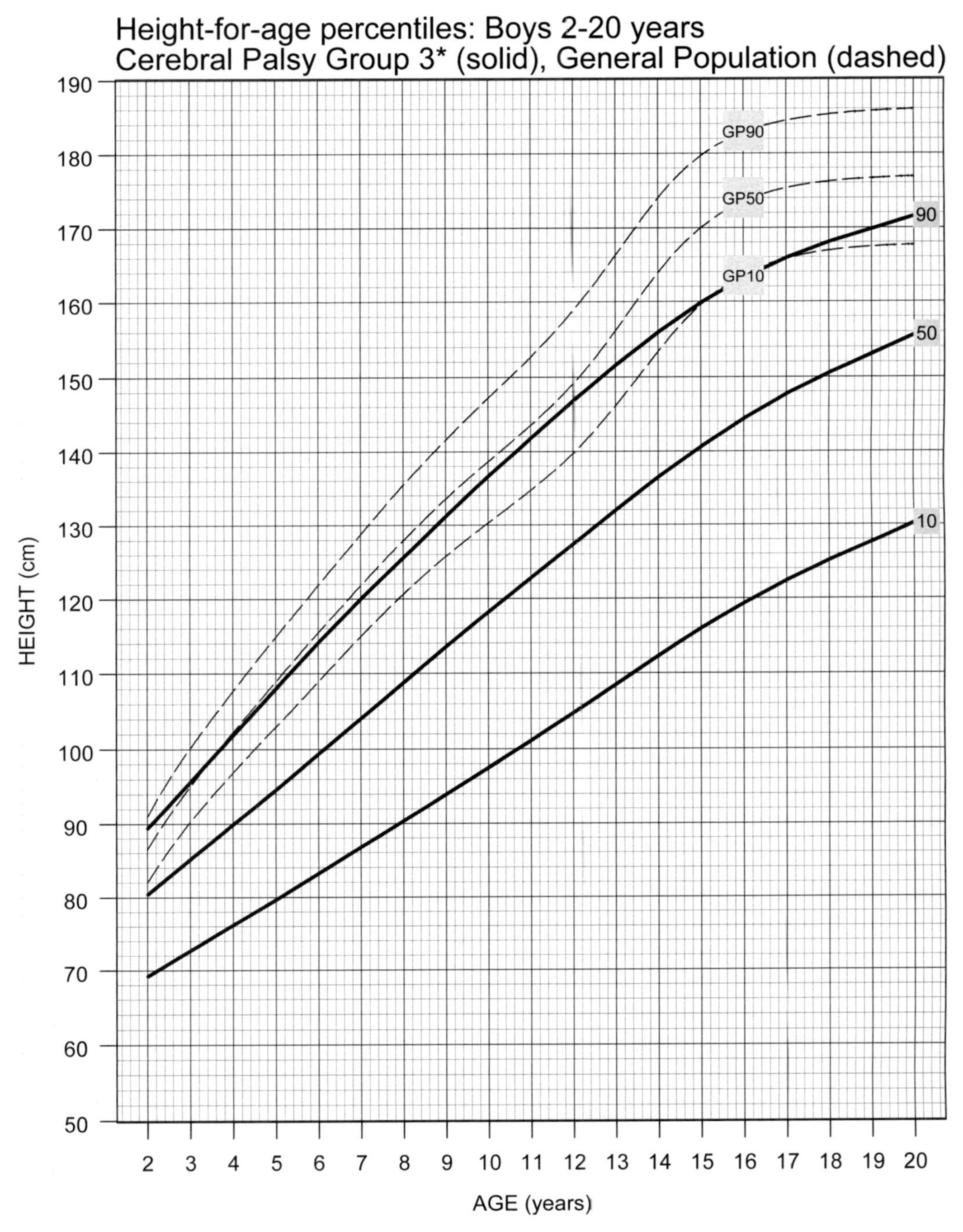

*Group 3: Crawls, creeps or scoots, but does not walk.

Appendix 1 ix

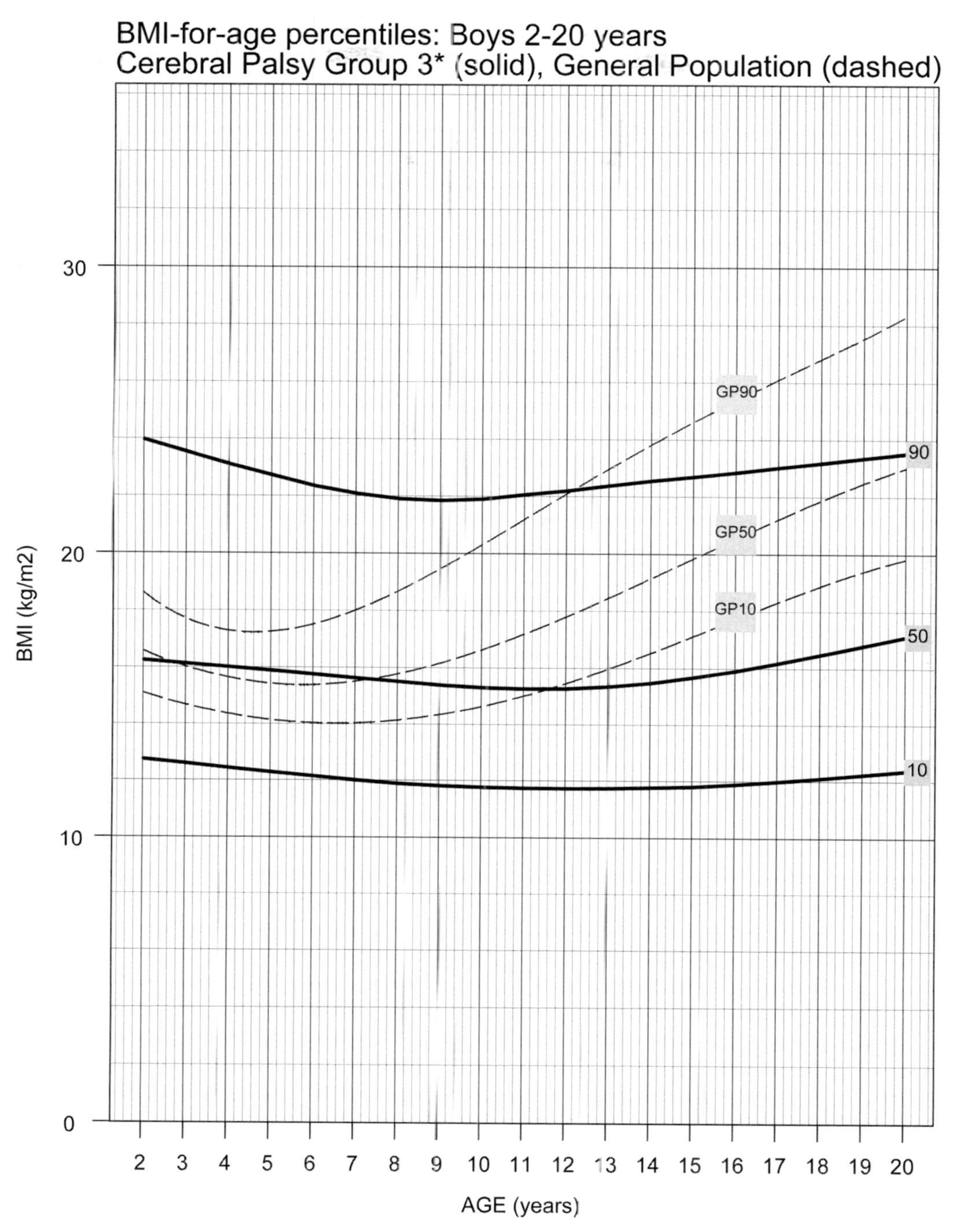

*Group 3: Crawls, creeps or scoots, but does not walk.

Appendix 1 x

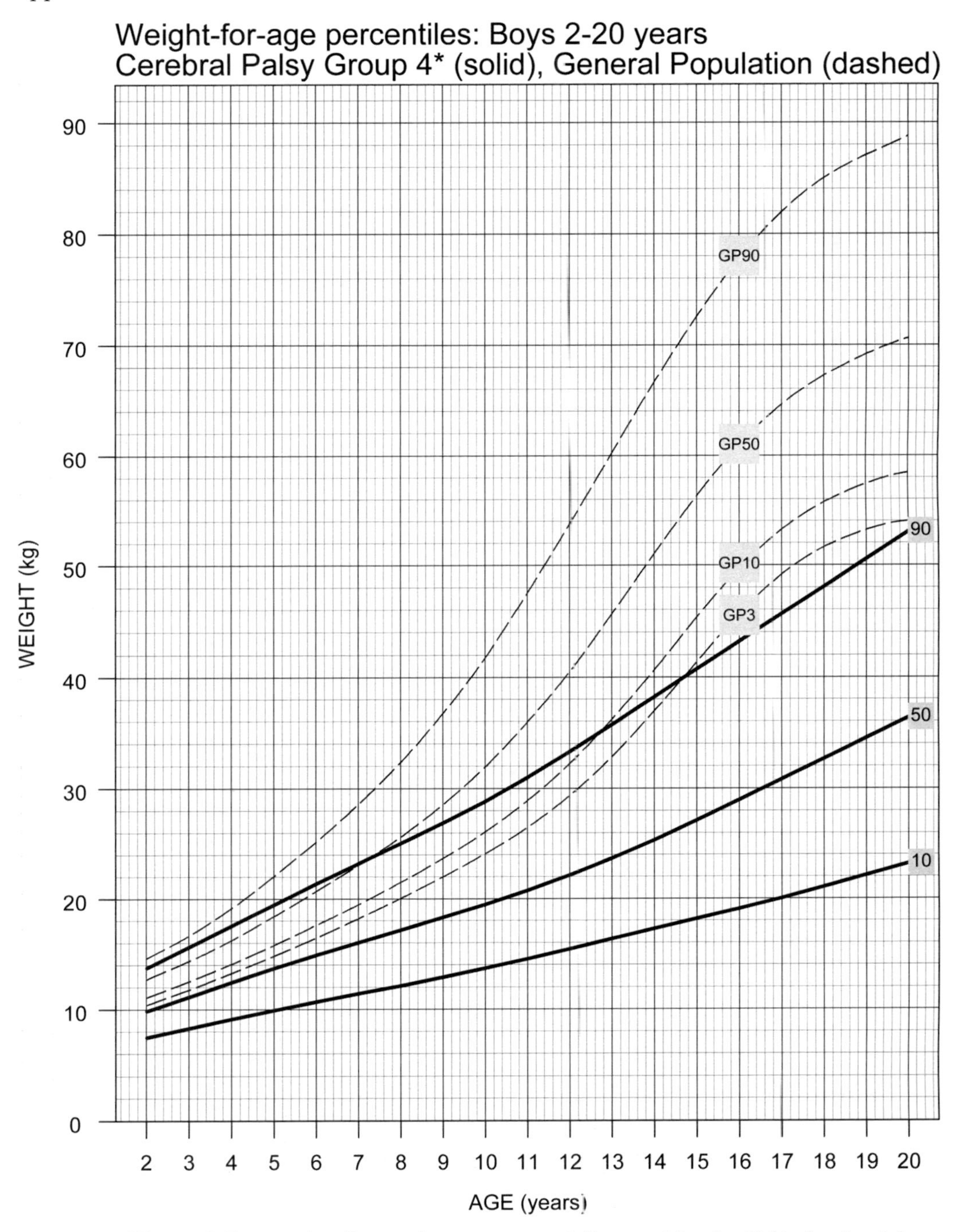
Weight-for-age percentiles: Boys 2-20 years
Cerebral Palsy Group 4* (solid), General Population (dashed)
WEIGHT (kg)
0
10
20
30
40
50
60
70
80
90
AGE (years)
2
3
4
5
6
7
8
9
10
11
12
13
14
15
16
17
18
19
20
GP90
GP50
GP10
GP3
90
50
10
*Group 4: Does not walk, crawl, creep or scoot; Does not feed self; No feeding tube.

Appendix 1 xi

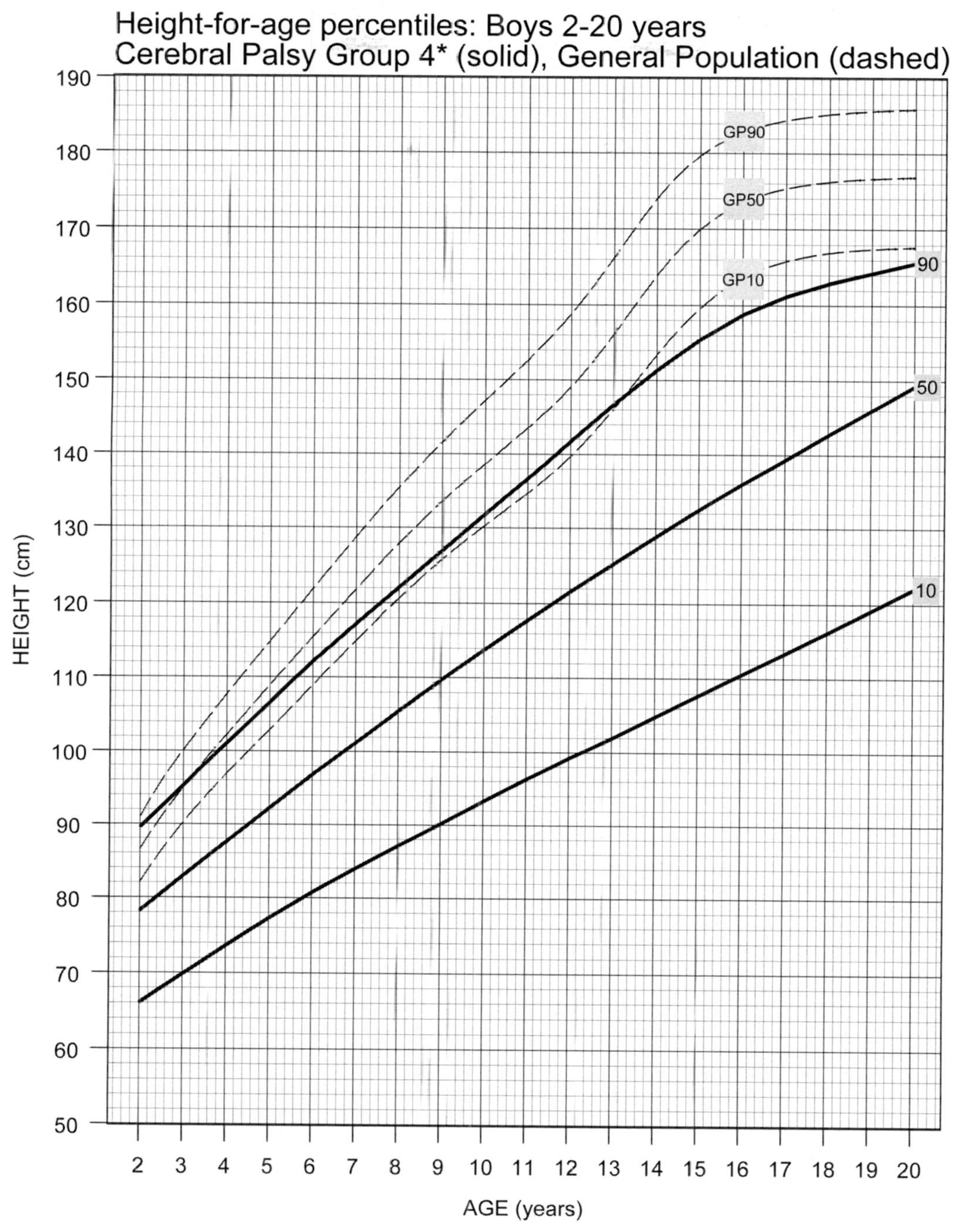

*Group 4: Does not walk, crawl, creep or scoot; Does not feed self; No feeding tube.

Appendix 1 xii

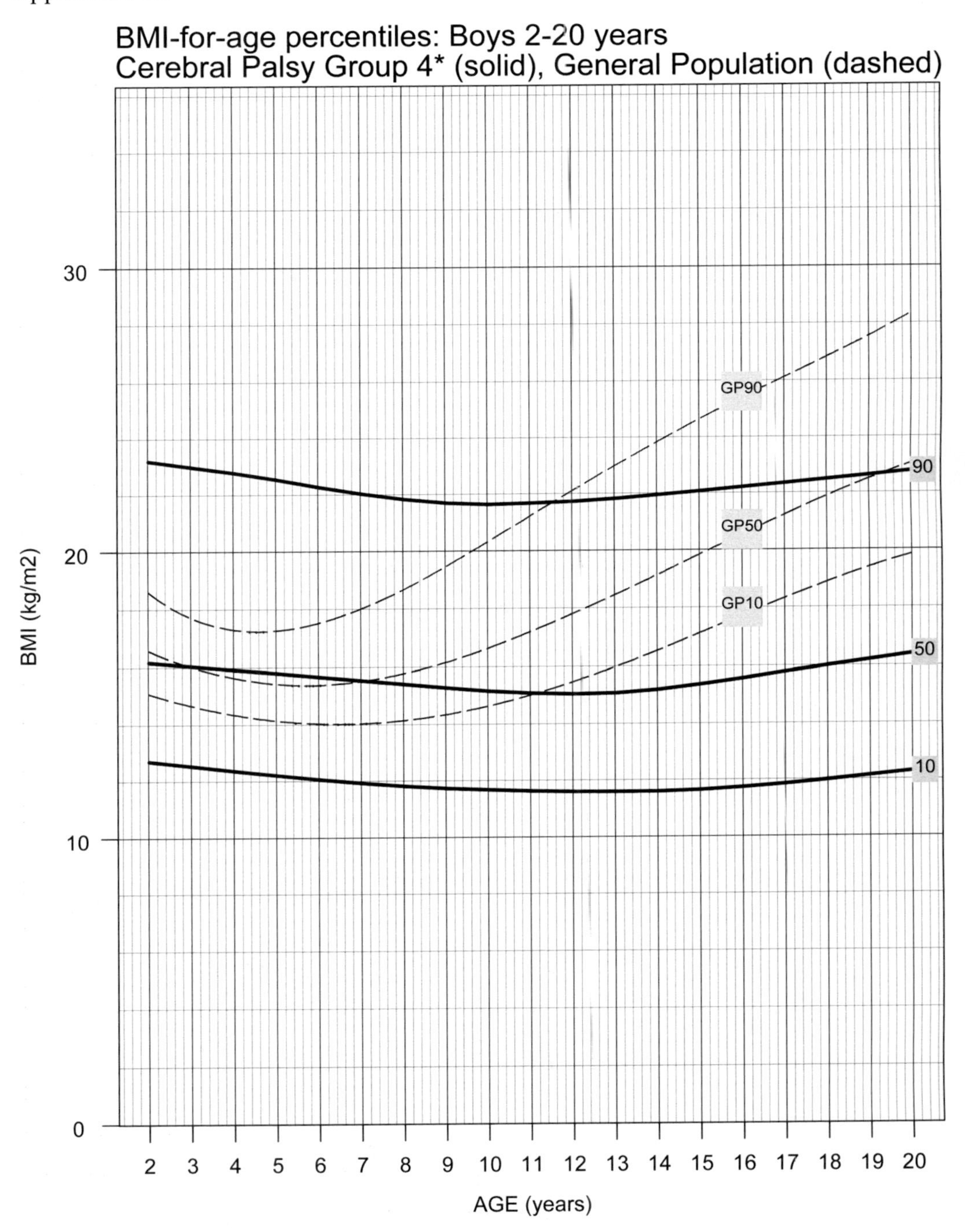

*Group 4: Does not walk, crawl, creep or scoot; Does not feed self; No feeding tube.

Appendix 1 xiii

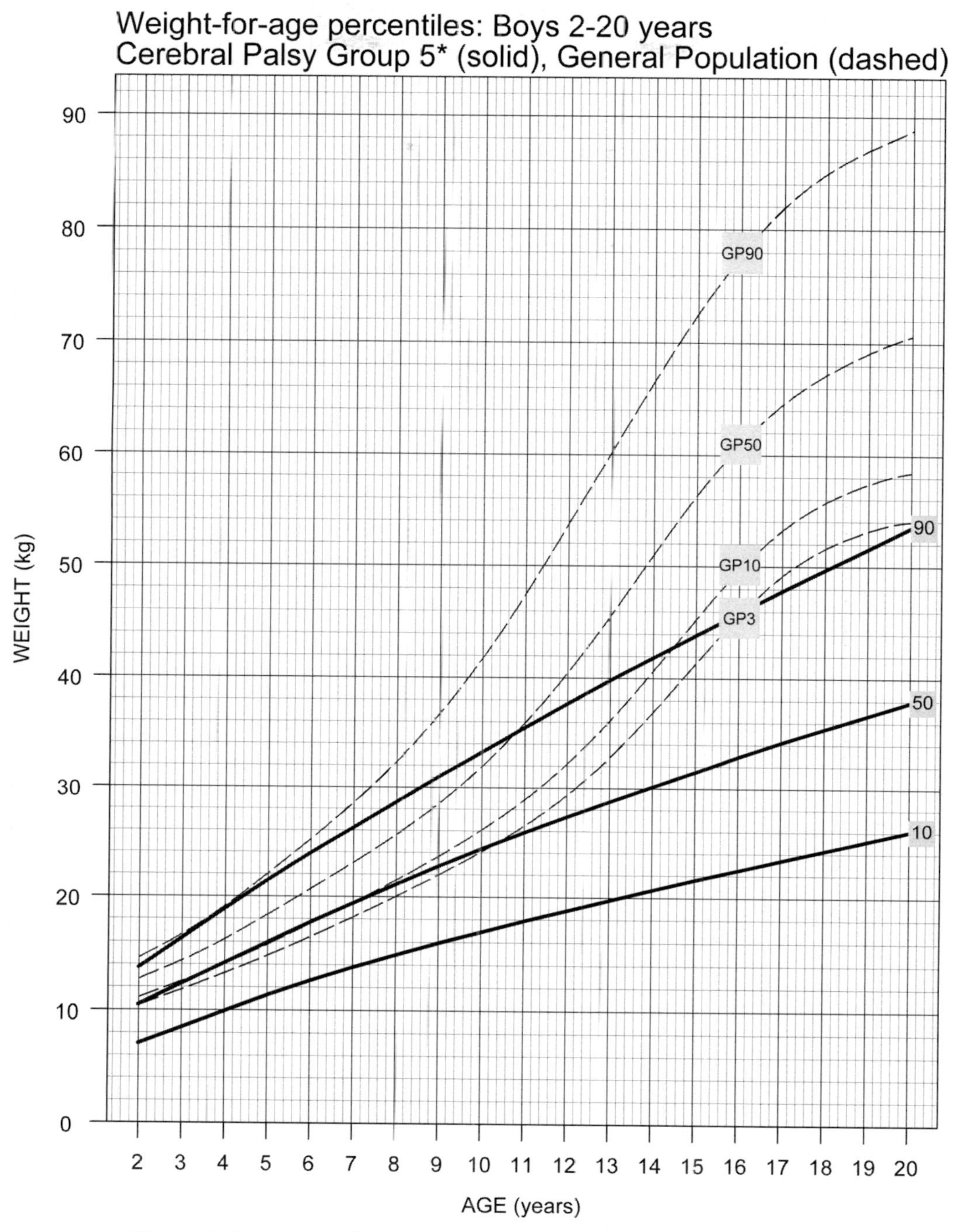

*Group 5: Does not walk, crawl, creep or scoot; Does not feed self; Feeding tube.

Appendix 1 xiv

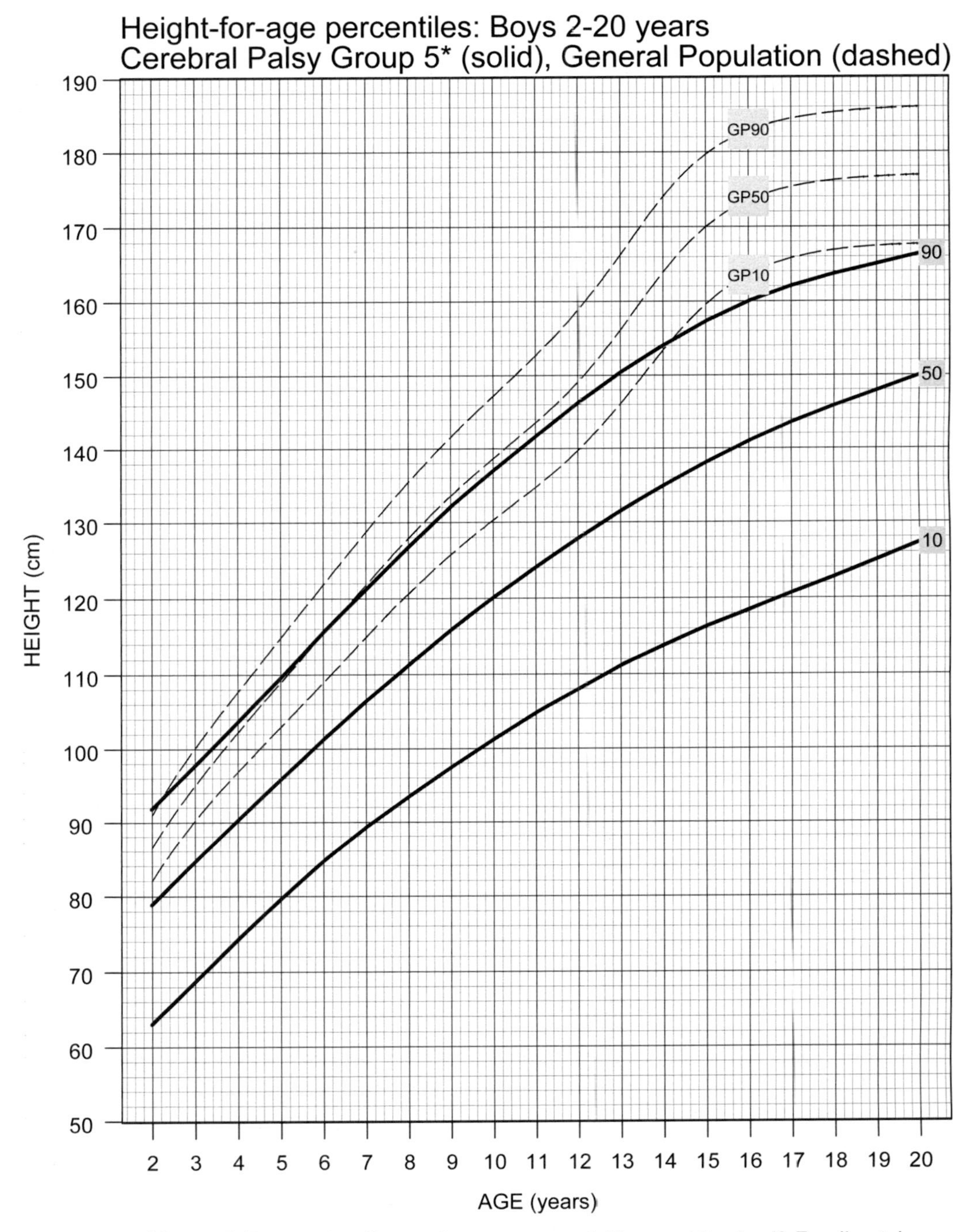

Appendix 1 xv

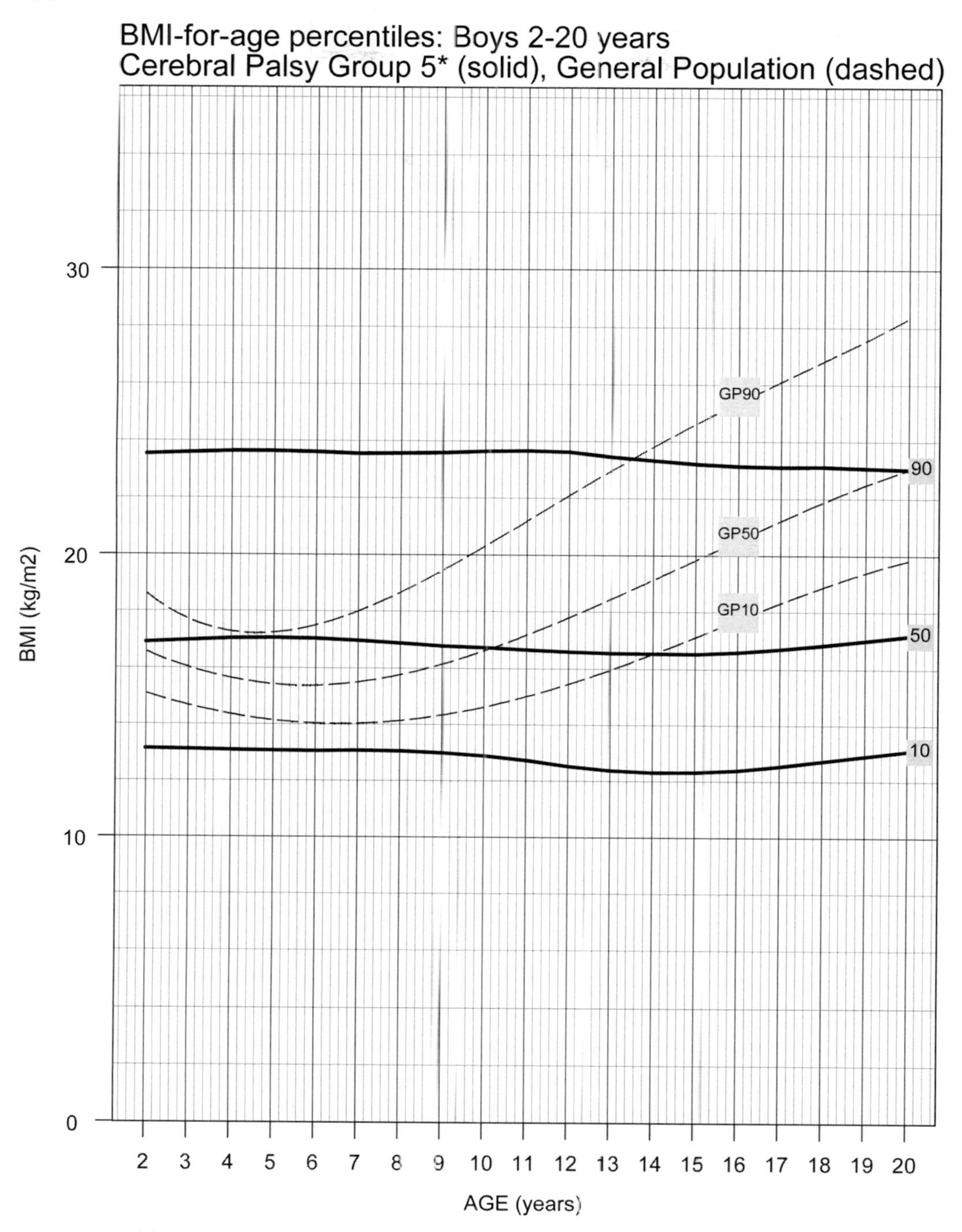

*Group 5: Does not walk, crawl, creep or scoot; Does not feed self; Feeding tube.

Appendix 1 xvi

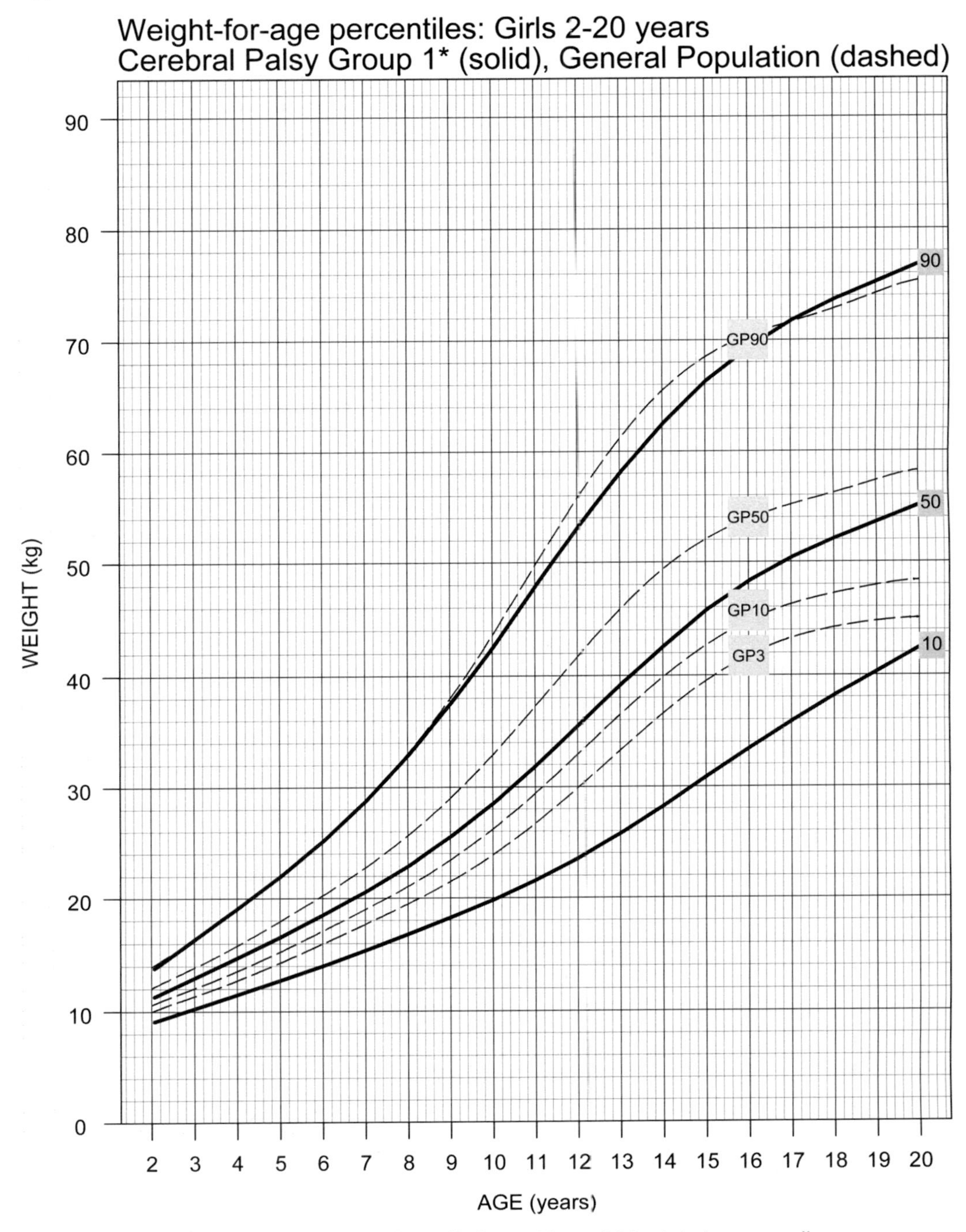

Appendix 1 xvii

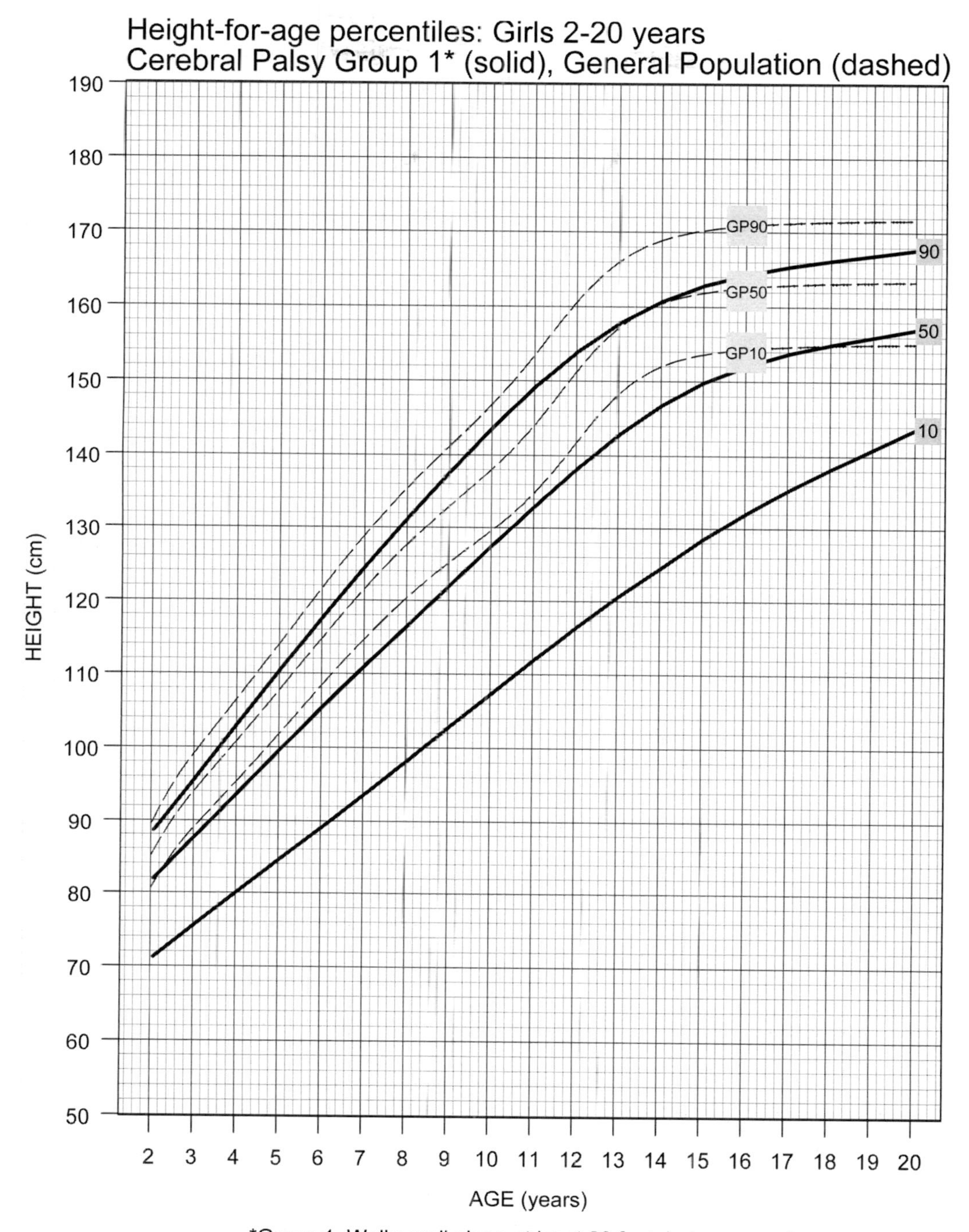

*Group 1: Walks well alone at least 20 feet, balances well.

Appendix 1 xviii

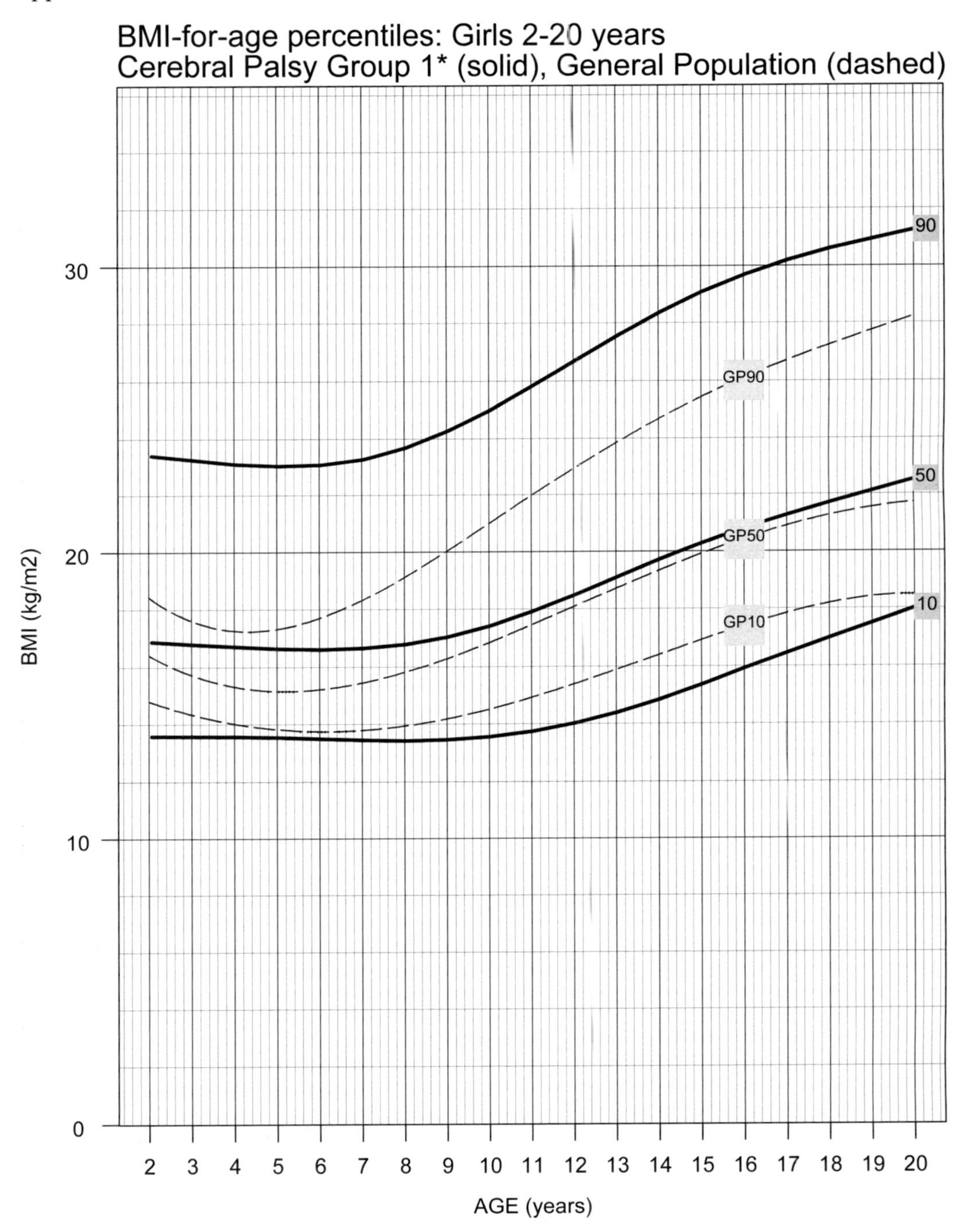

*Group 1: Walks well alone at least 20 feet, balances well.

Appendix 1 xix

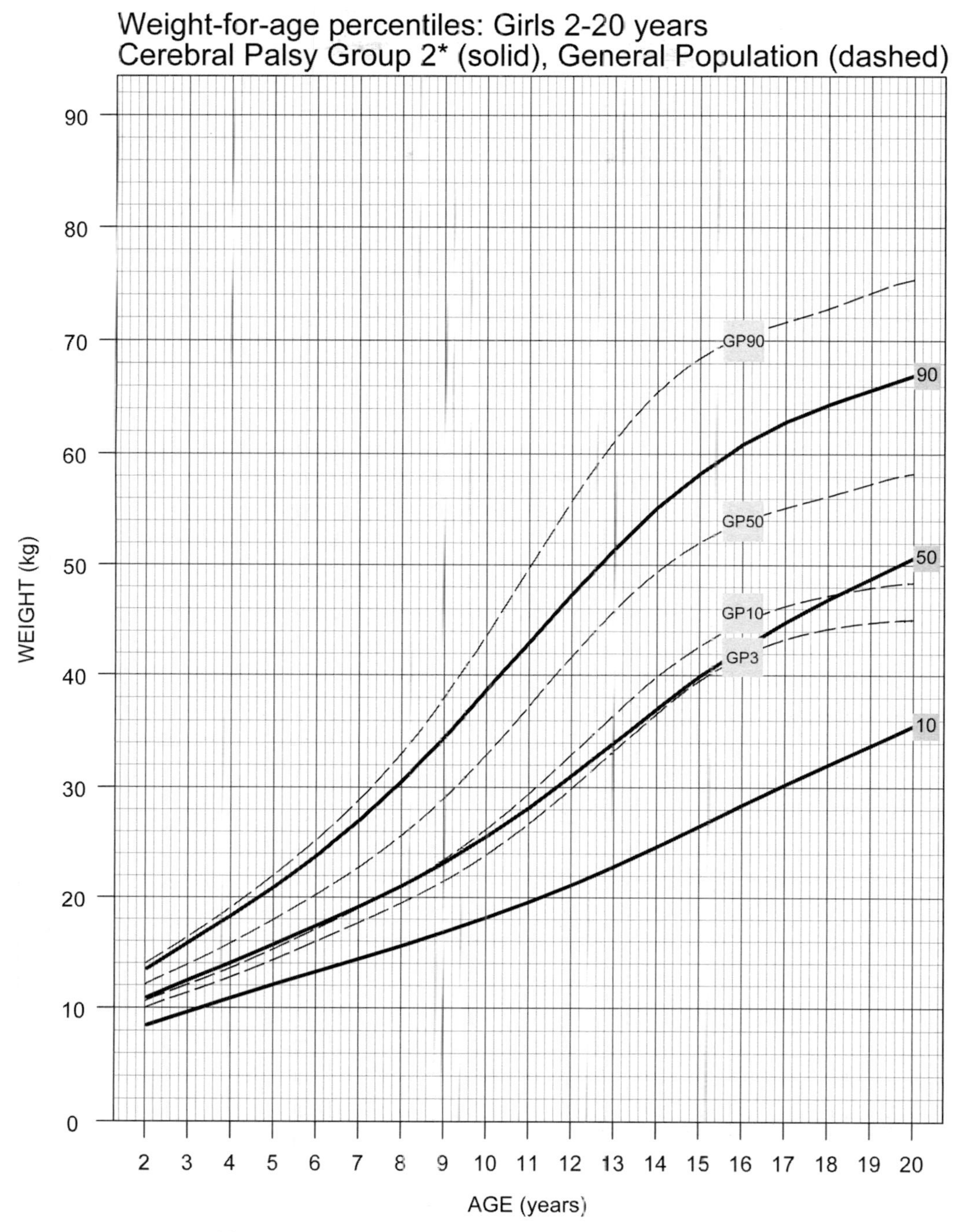

*Group 2: Walks with support or unsteadily alone at least 10 feet.

Appendix 1 xx

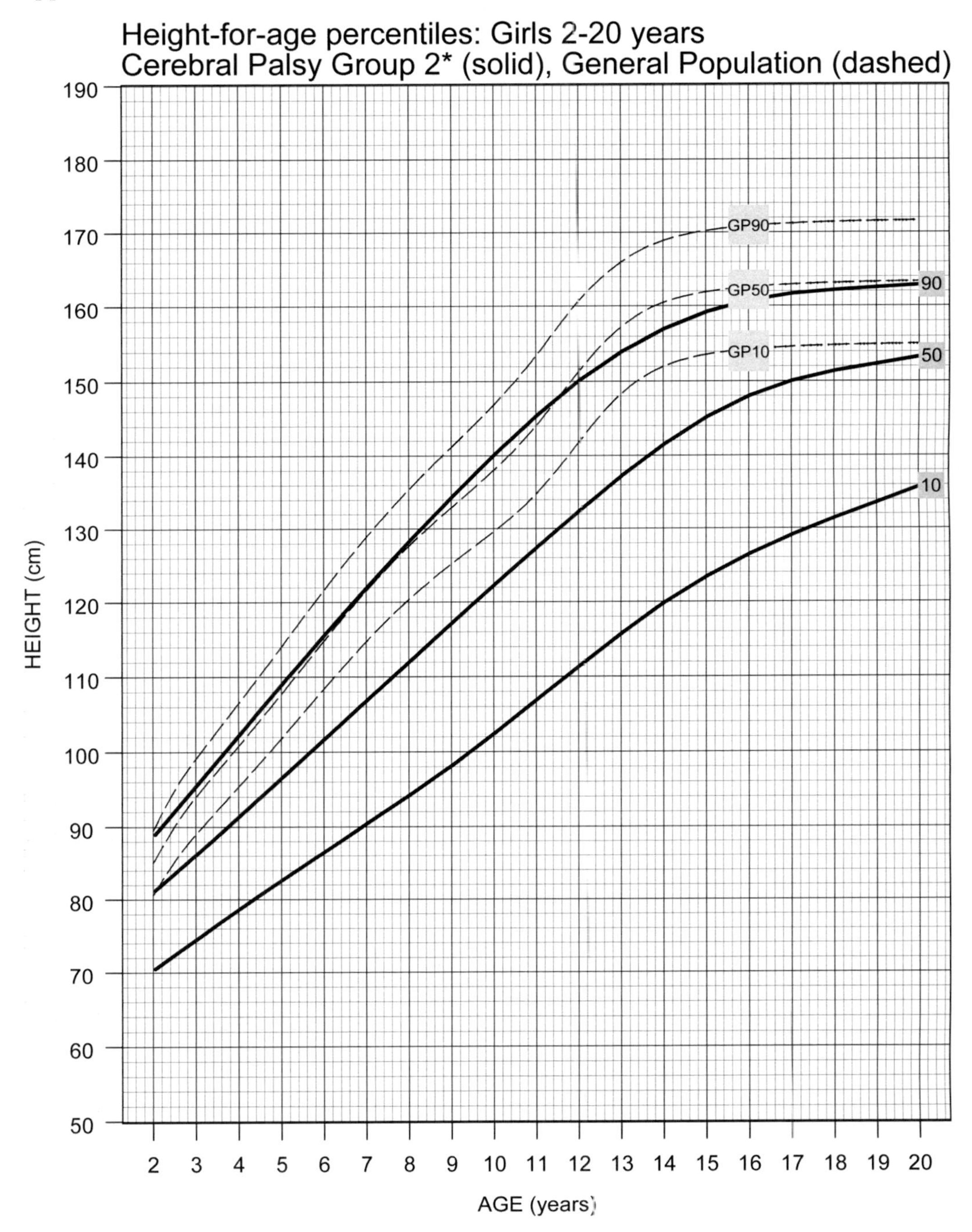

*Group 2: Walks with support or unsteadily alone at least 10 feet.

Appendix 1 xxi

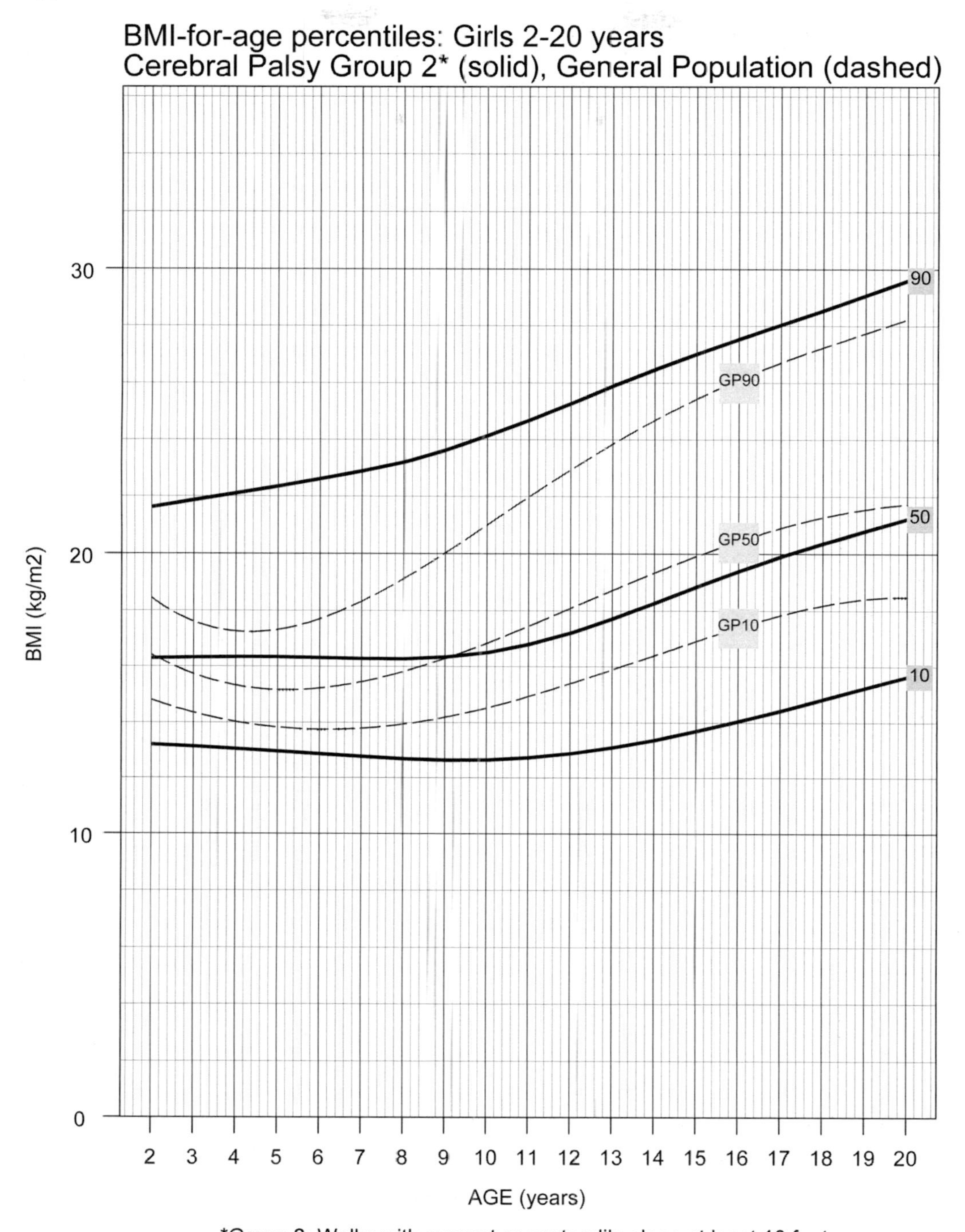

*Group 2: Walks with support or unsteadily alone at least 10 feet.

Appendix 1 xxii

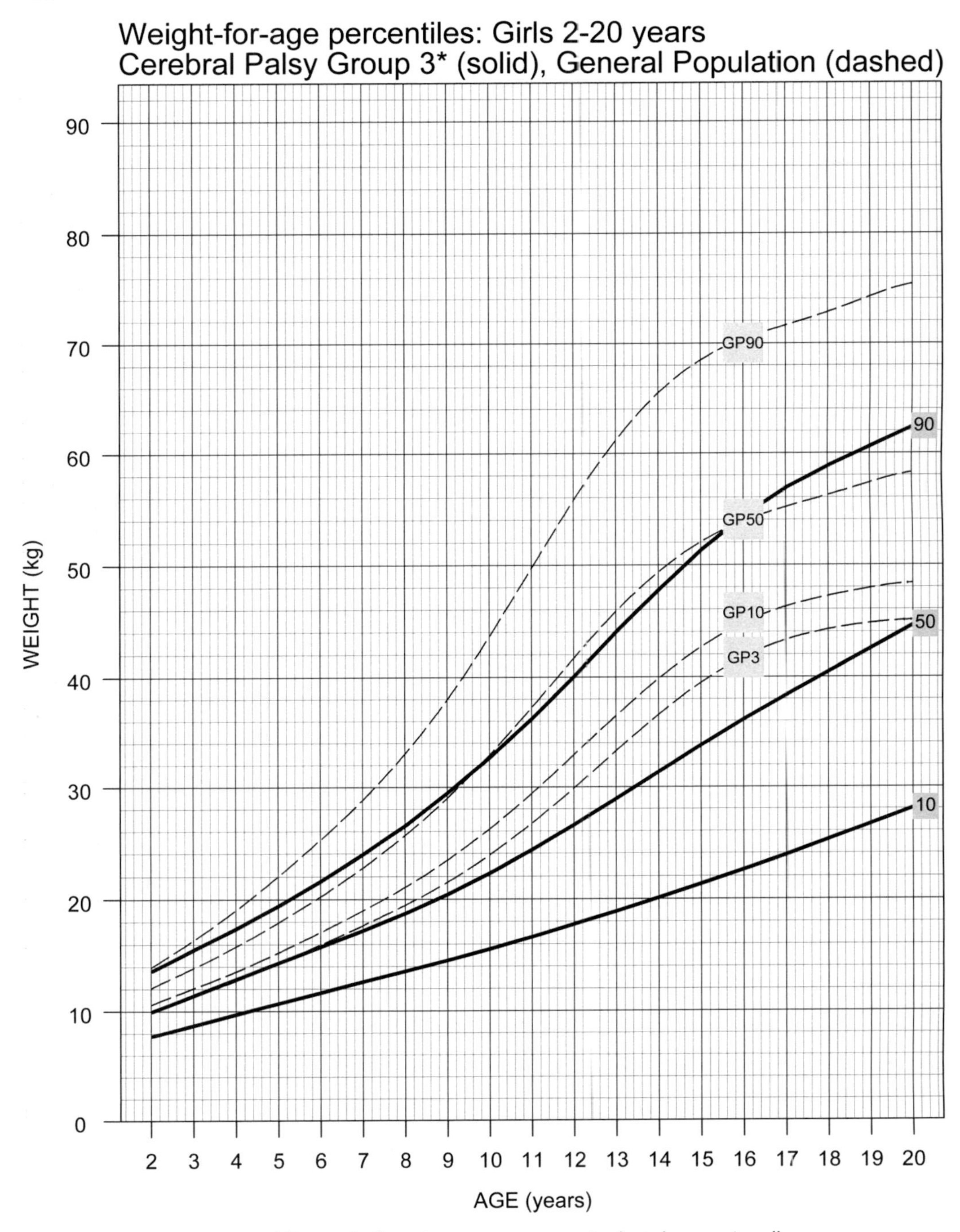

*Group 3: Crawls, creeps or scoots, but does not walk.

Appendix 1 xxiii

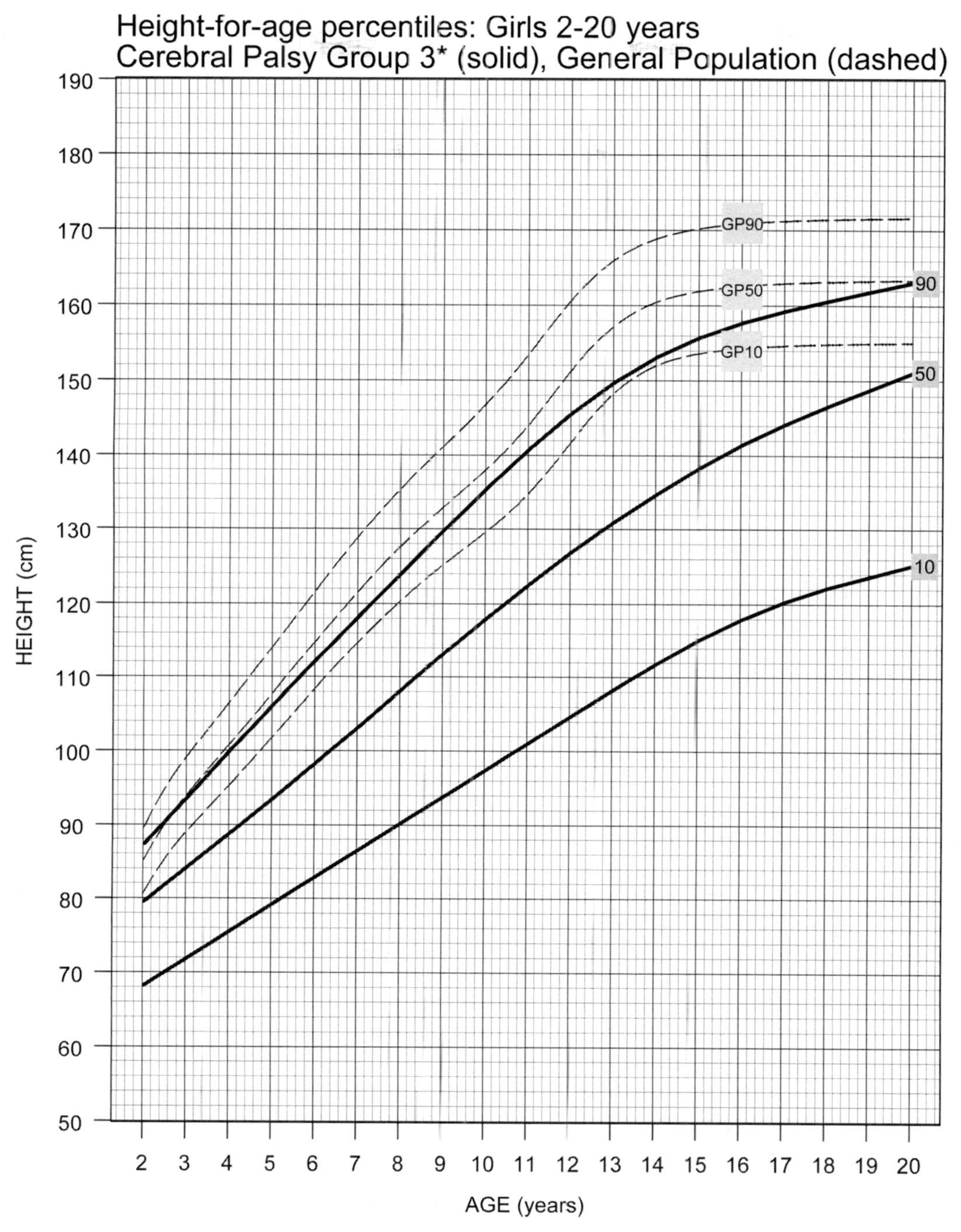

*Group 3: Crawls, creeps or scoots, but does not walk.

Appendix 1 xxiv

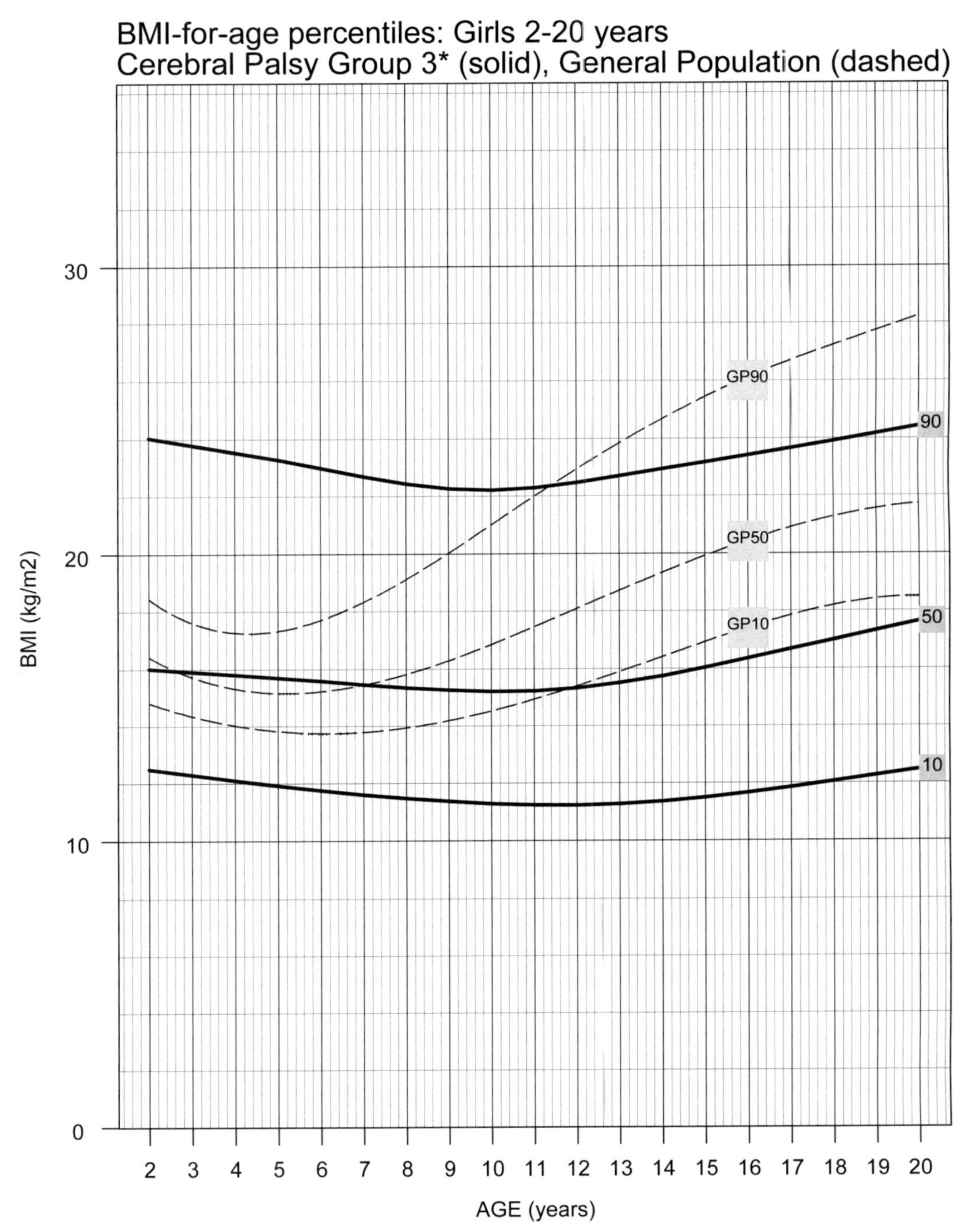

*Group 3: Crawls, creeps or scoots, but does not walk.

Appendix 1 xxv

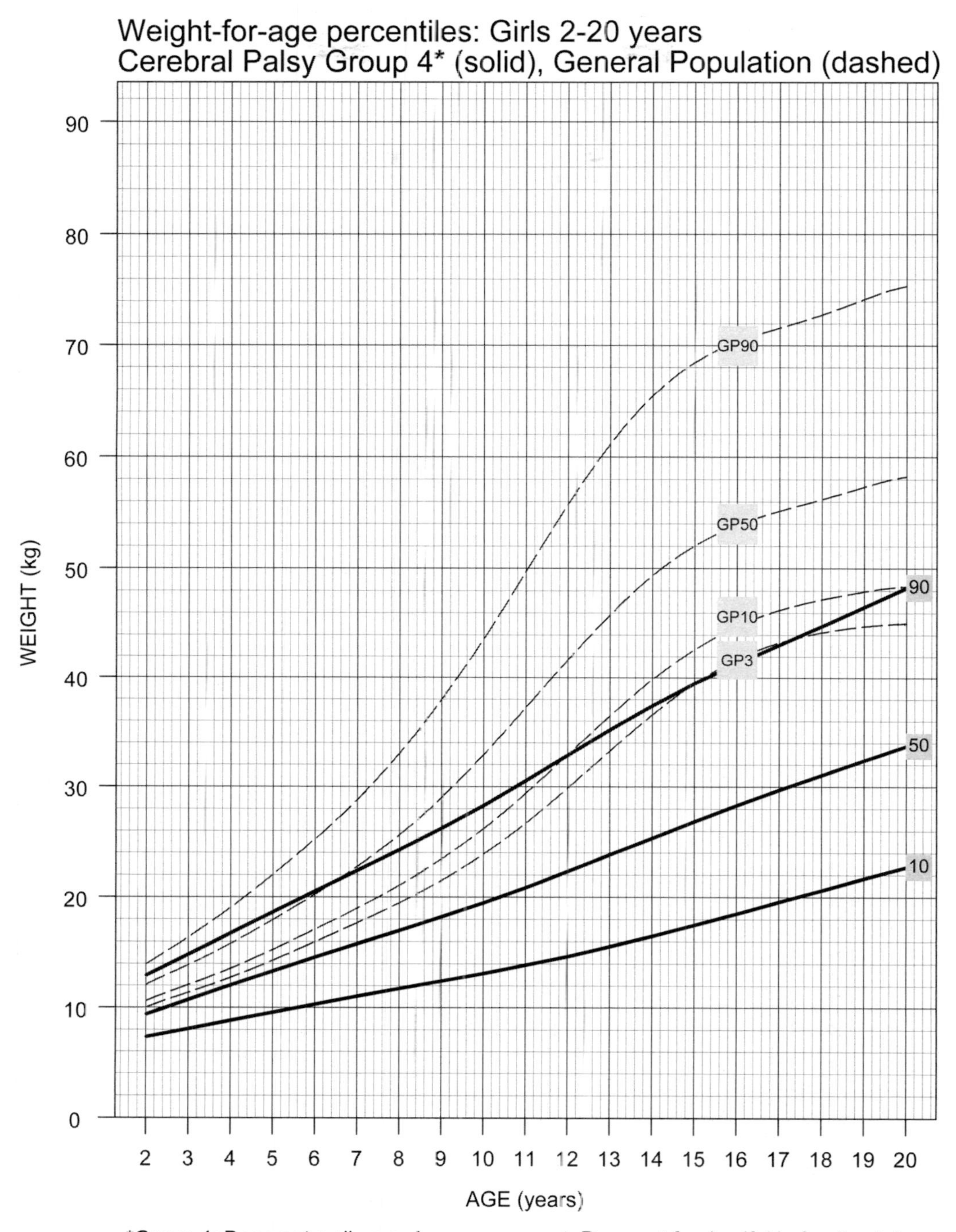

*Group 4: Does not walk, crawl, creep or scoot; Does not feed self; No feeding tube.

Appendix 1 xxvi

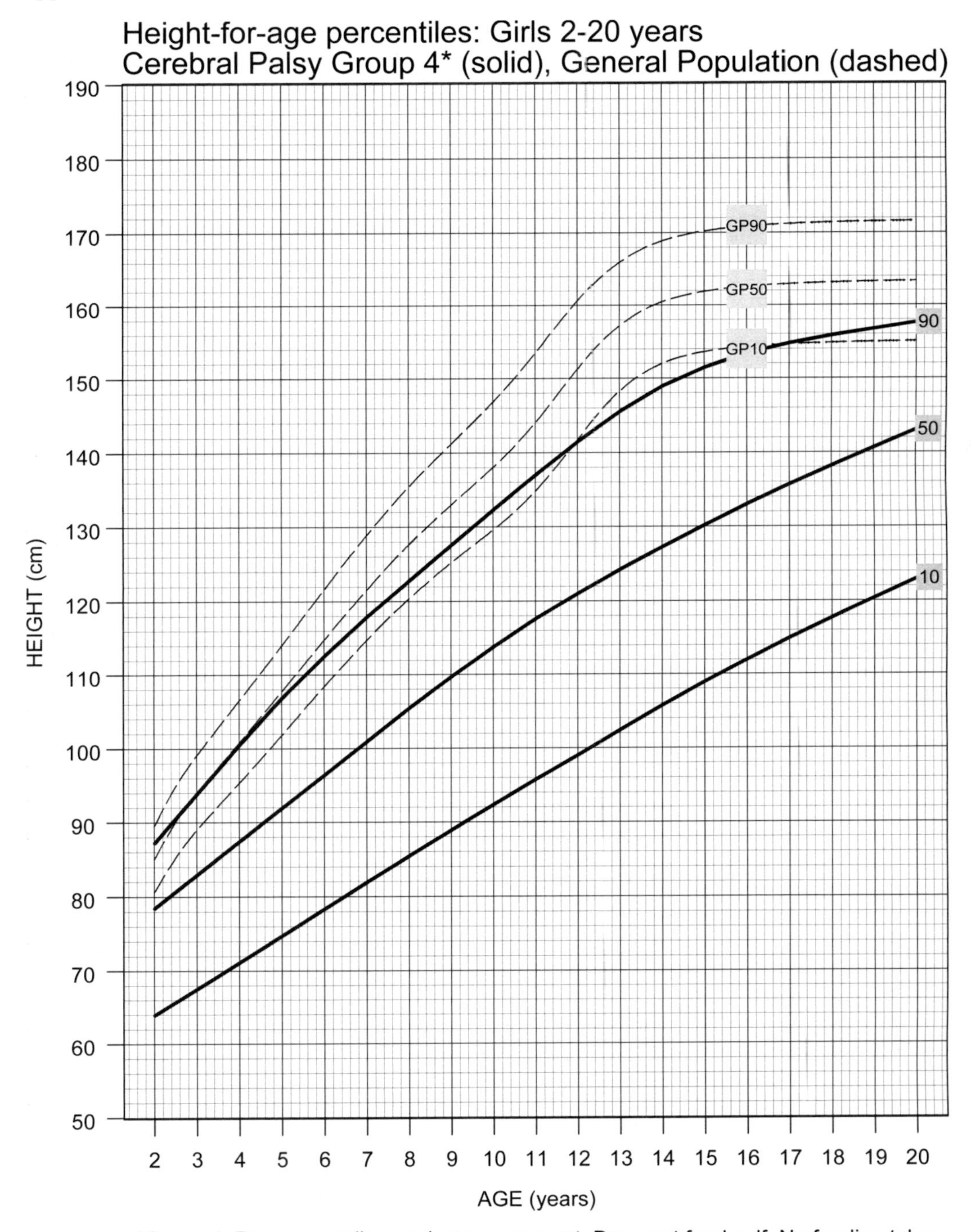

*Group 4: Does not walk, crawl, creep or scoot; Does not feed self; No feeding tube.

Appendix 1 xxvii

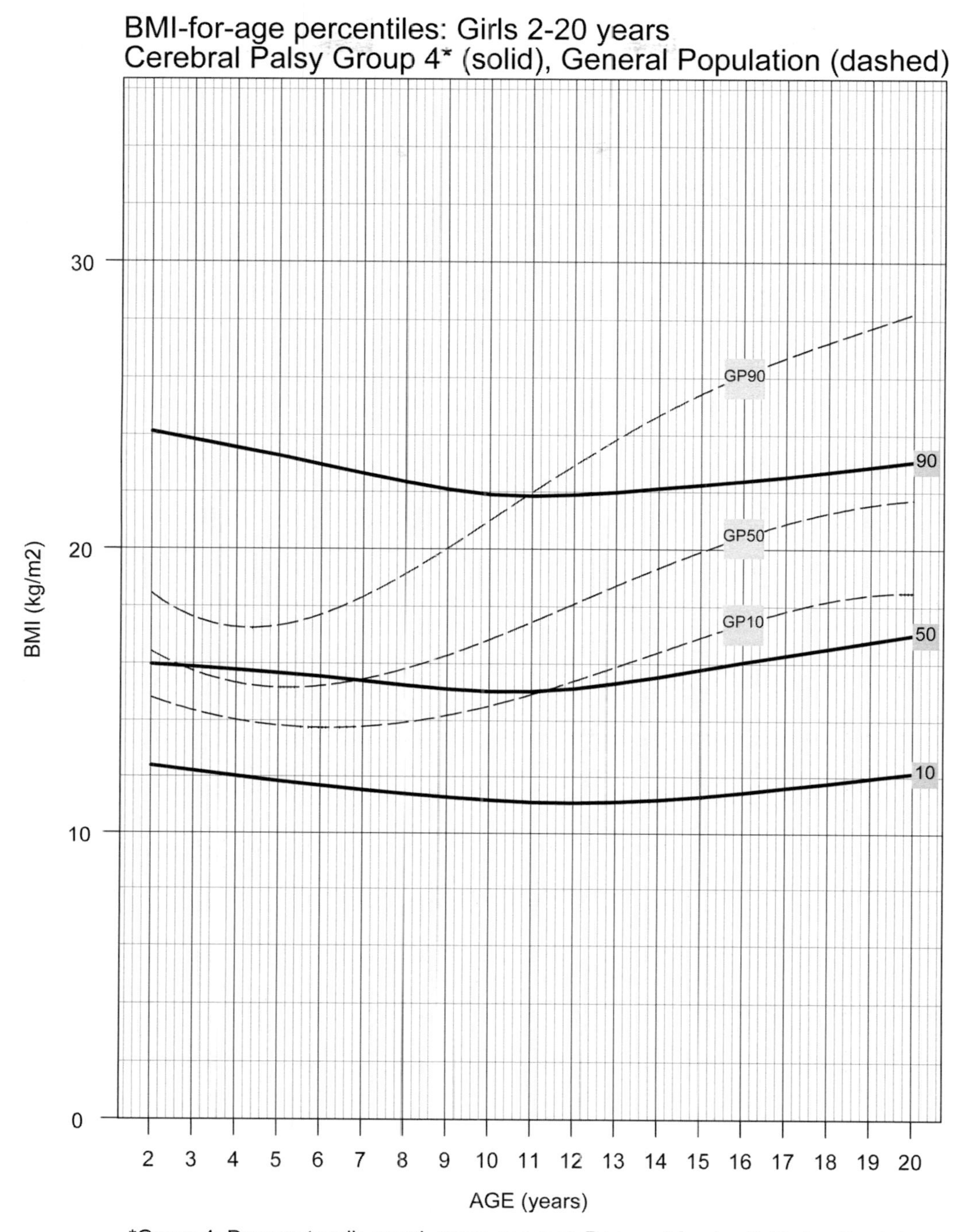

*Group 4: Does not walk, crawl, creep or scoot; Does not feed self; No feeding tube.

Appendix 1 xxviii

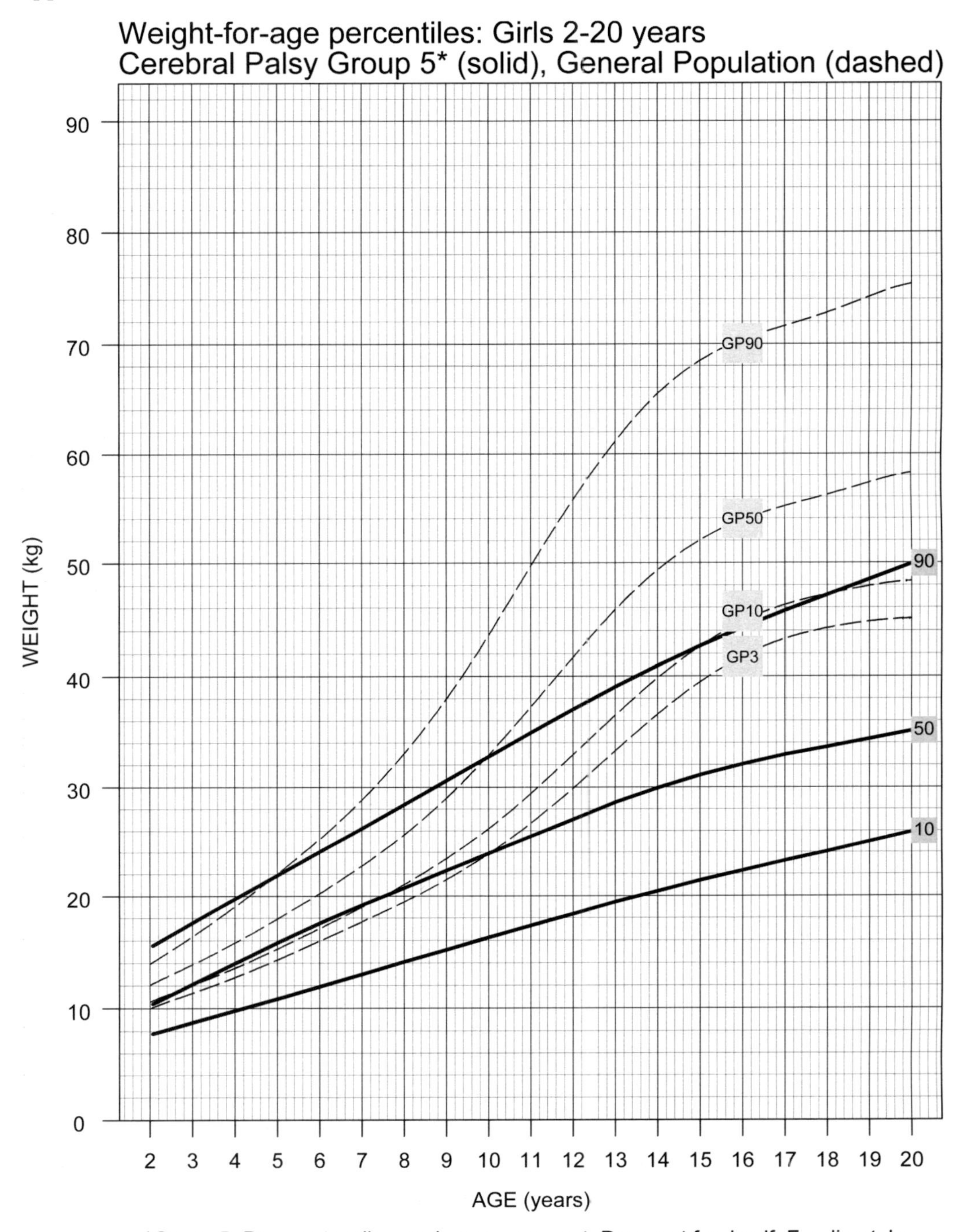

*Group 5: Does not walk, crawl, creep or scoot. Does not feed self; Feeding tube.

Appendix 1 xxix

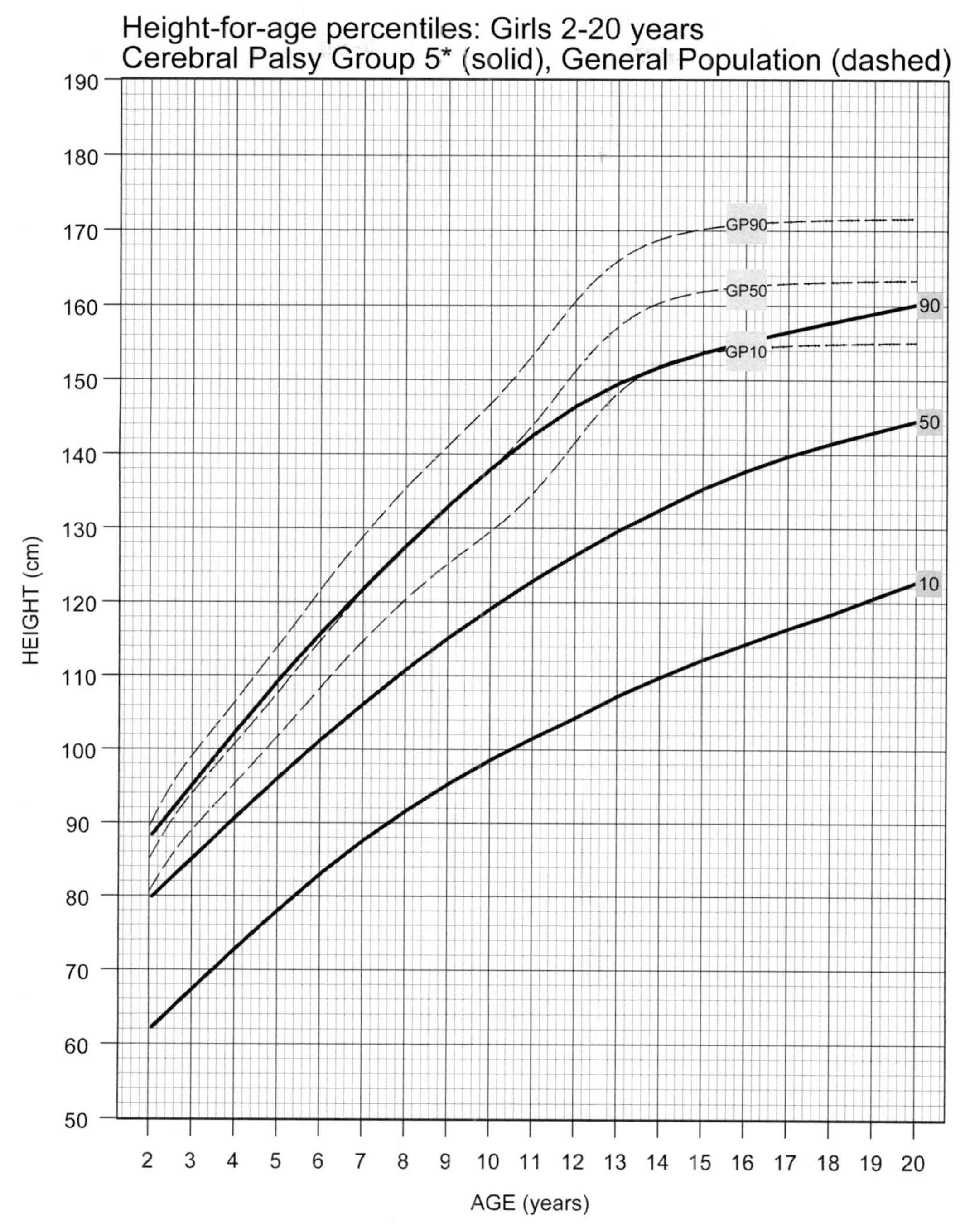

*Group 5: Does not walk, crawl, creep or scoot; Does not feed self; Feeding tube.

Appendix xxx

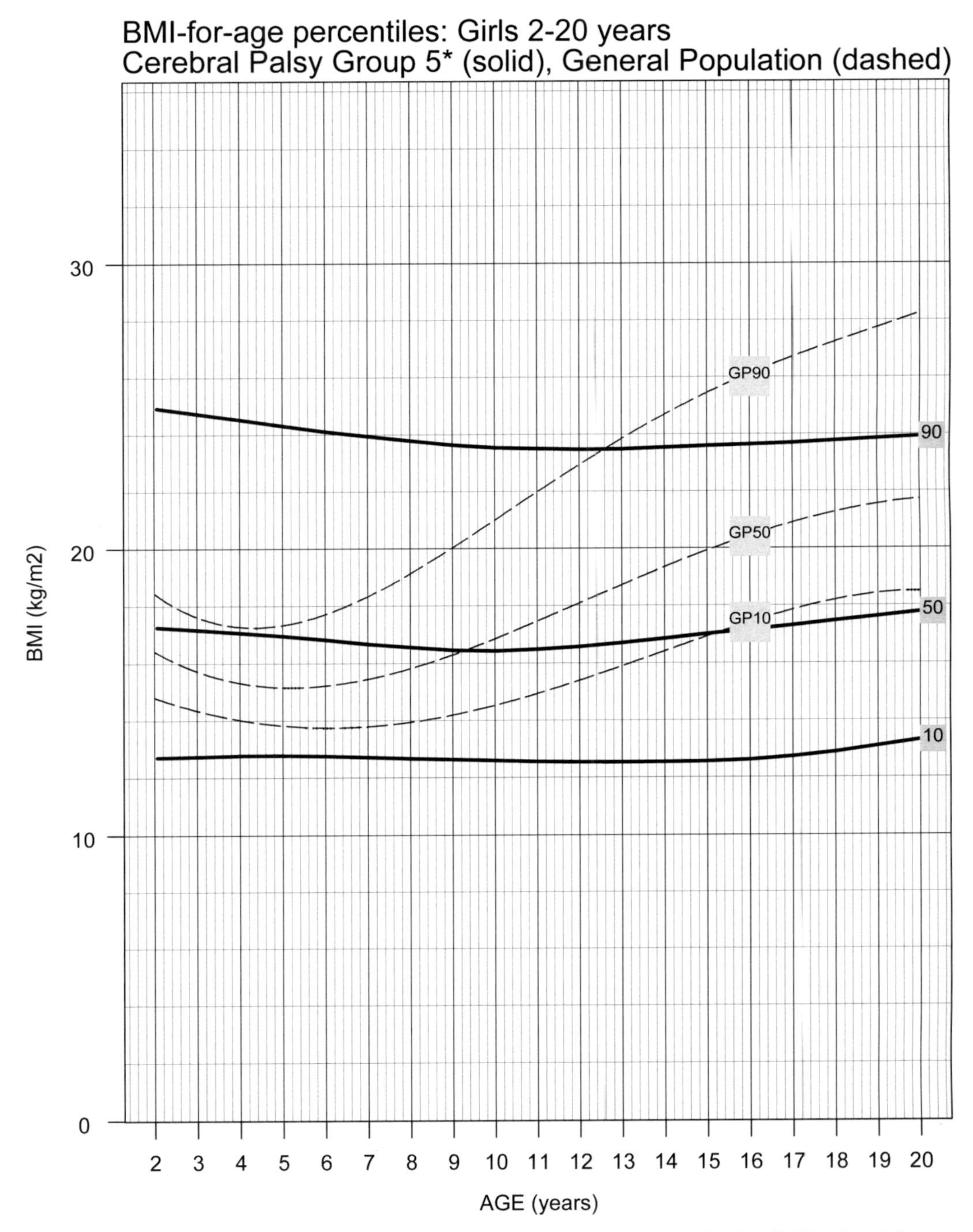

*Group 5: Does not walk, crawl, creep or scoot; Does not feed self; Feeding tube.

Appendix 2: Useful contacts and websites

Enteral nutrition
American Society for Parenteral and Enteral Nutrition (ASPEN)
http://www.nutritioncare.org/

British Association of Parenteral and Enteral Nutrition (BAPEN)
http://www.bapen.org.uk/

Patients on Intravenous and Nasogastric Nutrition Therapy (PINNT)
http://www.pinnt.co.uk/

Parenteral and Enteral Nutrition Group
http://www.peng.org.uk/

Support
4 My Child
http://www.cerebralpalsy.org/

United Cerebral Palsy (UCP)
http://www.ucp.org/

SCOPE homepage
http://www.scope.org.uk/

Cerebra
http://www.cerebra.org.uk/

British Institute for Brain Injured Children
http://www.bibic.org.uk/

Contact a Family
http://www.cafamily.org.uk/

Family Fund
http://www.familyfund.org.uk/

Face 2 Face
http://www.face2facenetwork.org.uk/

Intervention planning
Occupational Therapy Direct
http://www.otdirect.co.uk/

Care Co-ordination Network UK
http://www.ccnuk.org.uk/

Dental Health
American Dental Association (ADA)
http://www.ada.org/

British Dental Health Foundation
http://www.dentalhealth.org.uk/

British Society for Disability and Oral Health
http://www.bsdh.org.uk/

Appendix 3: Nasogastric tube and gastrostomy tube care guidelines

Nasogastric tube care guidelines

CARE OF THE TUBE

- Checking position:
  - this should be done before anything is administered via the nasogastric tube;
  - wash and dry hands;
  - explain to the child what you are about to do;
  - use a 50 ml syringe to draw back a small amount of fluid from the stomach;
  - check the acidity of this fluid using Universal paper – the acidity should be pH 4 or less;
  - if it is not possible to aspirate fluid, either:
    - lie the child on their side and try again,
    - where possible, ask the child to drink a small amount of fluid and try to draw back after a few minutes,
    - if you are still unable to aspirate fluid contact the community or hospital team in charge of the child.

- Flushing tube:
  - always use a 50ml syringe when flushing the tube;
  - flush at least 3 times a day with boiled, cooled water;
  - always flush after giving feed or medications with 5–10 ml of boiled, cooled water.

- Skin care:
  - for long term use apply a barrier product (e.g. hydrocolloid dressings) to the skin and fasten the tube with a transparent dressing on top;
  - alternate nostrils where possible to protect skin integrity.

COMMON PROBLEMS AND SOLUTIONS

What to do in an emergency

- If, during feeding, the child experiences any of the following symptoms STOP the feed and seek medical attention if they do not recover immediately:
  - sudden pallor,
  - shortness of breath,
  - vomiting,
  - coughing;

- If the tube is pulled out part of the way:
  - do not put anything down the tube unless the correct position has been confirmed,
  - do not try and replace the tube unless you have received the correct training,
  - remove the tube all the way and contact the community or hospital team to replace the tube if appropriate;

- If the tube is pulled out all of the way:
  - do not try and replace the tube unless you have received the correct training,
  - contact the hospital or community team to replace the tube.

FEEDING

- Feed: the type, volume and times of feeds will be determined by the dietitian. This information should be provided for parents, carers, school and respite care.
- Contacts: telephone numbers for suppliers of feed and equipment should be kept at home, at school and at respite care.
- Changes: notify parent, carers, school and respite care immediately if any changes are made to the feeding plan.

CONTACTS

- Contact numbers for the hospital and community teams should be kept with the child at all times in case of emergency.

Gastrostomy tube care guidelines

CARE OF THE TUBE

- Daily care:
  - wash and dry hands before and after contact with the gastrostomy;
  - rotate the tube 360° daily;
  - flush the tube with boiled, cooled water before and after giving feeds and medications, and at least once a day if not in use;
  - observe the site daily for changes in appearance which could indicate an infection.

- Hygiene:
  - wash gastrostomy tube site daily with boiled, cooled water;
  - clean daily with gauze or cotton buds, and with soap once the site has healed;
  - dry thoroughly and do not apply dressings to the site;

- Balloon:
  - check the water in the balloon after 2 weeks and then as required;
  - the gastrostomy tube will last varying amounts of time according to device type.

- Bathing and swimming:
  - the child can have a bath 10–14 days after the surgery provided the site has healed;
  - the child may shower 7 days after the operation;
  - the child can go swimming after 4 weeks, provided the site has healed;
  - apply a waterproof dressing to cover the tube;
  - do not allow swimming if the site is inflamed or the skin broken.

Common problems and solutions

- If, during feeding, the child experiences any of the following symptoms STOP the feed and seek medical attention if they do not recover immediately:
  - sudden pallor;
  - shortness of breath;
  - vomiting;
  - Coughing.

- If the tube is pulled out:
  - the child should have with them at all times a syringe, spigot, tape and Foley catheter;
  - as soon as the tube is out insert the Foley catheter up to 5 cms into the gastrointestinal tract;
  - inflate the balloon with 5 ml of air;
  - insert the spigot and secure with tape;
  - fix the Foley catheter in place to the skin using the tape;
  - do not use the tube for feeding until you have consulted the community team;
  - seek help from the community or hospital team for replacement of the gastrostomy.

- Infection/granulation:
  - if the site is red, sore, discharging, or smells unusual, contact the community team immediately;
  - if granulation tissue is noticed seek help from the community team. An antibiotic or steroid cream will be prescribed to apply to the site.

- Blockages:
  - if the tube appears blocked try flushing with warm water;
  - if the blockage persists try purging the tube using gentle pressure with 10–15 ml of pineapple juice or flat coke.

FEEDING

- Feed: type, volume and times of feed should be provided for parents, carers, school and respite care.
- Contacts: telephone numbers for suppliers of feed and equipment should be kept at home, at school and at respite care.
- Changes: notify parent, carers, school and respite care immediately if any changes are made to the feeding plan.

CONTACTS

- Contact numbers for the hospital and community teams should be kept with the child at all times in case of emergency.

Appendix 4: Incorporating nutrient-dense foods into the diet of children with feeding problems

Food	Ways of incorporating into the diet
Red meat and poultry	Cook stews and casseroles longer than normal recipe until meat is soft and tears easily Use minced meat to reduce chewing effort
Fish	Flake and add to omelette/scrambled egg Mash finely and mix in with mash potatoes
Egg	Add to mince meat or fish as a binding agent to make meatballs Mix well into soft-boiled rice, well-cooked noodles or well-cooked pasta and do a quick stir-fry until cooked Add an extra egg yolk to omelette/scrambled egg Mash hard-boiled eggs into mash potatoes Dip soft bread without crust into beaten egg and fry until egg is cooked
Cheese	Grate and add solid cheeses to sauces and gravies for potatoes, pasta, vegetables and meat Hard cheese like parmesan cheese can be finely grinded and sprinkled over mash potatoes and well-cooked pasta
Cream cheese	Boil potatoes and mash the potatoes on their own before adding the cream cheese and some milk or cream Stir through creamy pasta sauce to thicken Stir into scrambled eggs as they are cooking Mix with some honey, maple syrup, jam or icing sugar, sprinkle crushed biscuits over and serve as a dessert Soft cheese cubes/triangles can be given as between meals snacks
Tofu	Add cubed tofu to casseroles and soups Substitute part of ricotta cheese in recipes like lasagne or ravioli with mashed tofu Blend tofu with fruits to make smoothies Use tofu in mousse or cheesecake recipes
Beans, e.g. black eye beans, pinto beans	Mash and mix into mash potatoes Add to casseroles and soups
Mushrooms	Chop and add to casseroles, soups and sauces Grilled mushrooms can be sliced and used as sandwich or jacket potato fillers
Nuts (if no allergy and choking is not a risk)	Chopped nuts can be tossed into pasta, rice and noodles Top ice cream and yogurt with chopped nuts Use ground hazelnuts or almonds to flavour milk and porridge Smooth peanut butter can be spread on soft bread without crusts Other nuts can be blended with oil to make nut butter and be used as a spread on soft bread without crusts

Food	Ways of incorporating into the diet
Liver	Marinate slices of liver in Japanese-style teriyaki sauce and grill or pan-fry Try liver pâté and spread on soft bread without crusts
Margarine/butter	Mix a dollop into just cooked vegetables, pasta, potatoes, rice Spread thicker layer on bread for sandwiches
Double cream	Add to milk with breakfast cereals or porridge Use to make sauces and soups Lightly whip double cream with icing sugar and serve with soft fruits or fruit purée
Orange-fleshed vegetables, e.g. carrots, sweet potatoes, butternut squash	Carrot juice can be mixed with orange juice and served as a drink with breakfast or other meals Purée or mash carrots, sweet potatoes and butternut squash with potatoes or on their own
Avocado	Use as a spread like butter, on bread Blend with milk to make a smoothie Chop and mix into mash potatoes Mix with cream cheese
Yeast/meat extract	Add to gravies and sauces Use as a marinade for meat before cooking
Wheat germ	Add to porridge or cereals Blend with milk powder, nuts and/or fruits to make a drink Use in home baked cakes or biscuits
Seeds, e.g. sesame seeds pumpkin seeds, sunflower seeds (larger seeds may need to be grinded to avoid choking incidents)	Spinkle over cereals and porridge Add to rice and pasta Use as topping for vegetable and meat dishes Use sesame seeds to make tahini and spread on bread in place of butter
Pine nuts (may need to be chopped/ grinded)	Use extra to make pesto; and pesto can be added to soups, sauces, pasta and vegetables Grind and sprinkle over soups and pasta
Wholemeal bread	Make into breadcrumbs and stir into gravies and sauces to thicken Use in place of or substitute half the quantity of white bread in pudding recipes, e.g. bread and butter pudding, summer pudding Dip in beaten egg and fry until egg is cooked, which will soften bread
Houmous	Spread on soft bread and top with other sandwich fillings, e.g. tuna, ham, egg
Miso (Japanese)	Use to make soup Use in dressings for salads, vegetables and fish

Appendix 5: Formula and supplement information

1. High energy infant formula

Product Name	Manufacturer	Nutritional composition per 100 ml												Osmolality (mOsmol/ kgH_2O)
		Energy (kcal)	Protein (g)	Fat (g)	Carb (g)	Fibre (g)	Lactose (g)	Vit A (μg RE)	Vit D (μg)	Calcium (mg)	Iron (mg)	Zinc (mg)	Selenium (μg)	
Infatrini	Nutricia	100	2.6	5.4	10.3	0	5.2	81	1.7	80	1.0	0.9	2.0	345
SMA High Energy	SMA Nutrition	91	2	4.9	9.8	-	9.8	100	1.4	57	1.1	0.8	1.9	415

2. Pre-thickened infant formula
These formulas thicken in the stomach in contact with gastric juices

Product Name	Manufacturer	Nutritional composition per 100 ml												Osmolality (mOsmol/ kgH_2O)
		Energy (kcal)	Protein (g)	Fat (g)	Carb (g)	Fibre (g)	Lactose (g)	Vit A (μg RE)	Vit D (μg)	Calcium (mg)	Iron (mg)	Zinc (mg)	Selenium (μg)	
Enfamil AR contains rice starch 2.1 g per 100 ml	Mead Johnson	68	1.7	3.5	7.6	0	4.3	60	1.0	55	0.7	0.7	1.5	230
SMA Staydown contains pre-cooked cornstarch 1.8g per 100ml	SMA Nutrition	67	1.6	3.6	7.0	0	5.0	75	1.1	56	0.8	0.6	1.4	246

3. Thickeners

Product Name	Manufacturer	Active ingredient	Lactose-free
Carobel	Cow & gate	Carob bean gum	No
Thicken Up	Nestle Nutrition	Pre-gelatinized waxy corn (maize) starch	Yes
Thick & Easy	Fresenius Kabi	Modified corn (maize) starch	Yes

4. Modular Supplements

Product name	Manufacturer	Type	Kcal
Super Soluble Duocal	SHS	Carbohydrate 73: Fat 22 powder	5 per gram
Procal shot liquid	Vitaflo	Protein, Fat and Carbohydrate emulsion from vegetable oil, skimmed milk powder, lactose and sodium caseinate	100 kcal 2 g protein per 30 ml shot
Super soluble Maxijul	SHS	Carbohydrate (Glucose polymer from maltodextrin) powder	4 per gram
Polycose	Abbott	Carbohydrate (Glucose polymer from hydrolysis of cornstarch) powder	4 per gram
Calogen	SHS	Fat emulsion of LCT	4.5 per ml

5. Polymeric (whole protein) formula

Product Name	Manu-facturer	Nutritional composition per 100 ml												Osmolality (mOsmol/ kgH_2O)
		Energy (kcal)	Protein (g)	Fat (g)	Carb (g)	Fibre (g)	Lactose (g)	Vit A (µg RE)	Vit D (µg)	Calcium (mg)	Iron (mg)	Zinc (mg)	Selenium (µg)	
Children aged 1–6 years or weight 8–20 kg														
Nutrini and Nutrini Multi Fibre	Nutricia	100	2.75	4.4	12.3	0.8[a]	<0.1	41	1.0	60	1.0	1.0	3.0	255
Nutrini Energy and Nutrini Energy Multi Fibre	Nutricia	150	4.1	6.7	18.5	0.8[a]	<0.1	61	1.5	90	1.5	1.5	4.5	415
Nutrini Low Energy Multi Fibre	Nutricia	75	2.1	3.3	9.3	0.8	<0.1	41	1.0	60	1.0	1.0	3.0	220
Children aged 1–10 years or weigh 8–30 kg														
Paediasure and Paediasure Fibre	Abbott	100	2.8	4.98	10.9	0.7[b]	0	45	1.0	56	1.0	1.0	2.8	340
Paediasure Plus and Paediasure Plus Fibre	Abbott	150	4.2	7.47	16.4	1.1[b]	0	99	1.1	83	1.5	1.5	4.2	347

5. Polymeric (whole protein) formula *continued*

Product Name	Manu-facturer	Nutritional composition per 100 ml												Osmolality (mOsmol/ kgH_2O)
		Energy (kcal)	Protein (g)	Fat (g)	Carb (g)	Fibre (g)	Lactose (g)	Vit A (µg RE)	Vit D (µg)	Calcium (mg)	Iron (mg)	Zinc (mg)	Selenium (µg)	
Children aged 7–12 years and above or weigh 21–45 kg														
Tentrini and Tentrini Multi Fibre	Nutricia	100	303	4.2	12.3	1.1[c]	<0.025	61	0.7	70	1.3	1.1	4.9	280
Tentrini Energy and Tentrini Energy Multi Fibre	Nutricia	150	4.9	6.3	18.5	1.1[c]	<0.025	92	1.1	95	2.0	1.7	7.4	430
Adult feeds – suitable for children aged 6 years and above														
Osmolite	Abbott	101	4.0	3.4	13.6	0	0	108	0.73	68	1.4	1.3	6.0	288
Jevity	Abbott	100	4.0	3.47	14.1	1.76	0	51.6	0.75	92	1.4	1.1	5.3	300
Jevity 1.5kcal	Abbott	152	6.38	4.9	20.1	2.2	0	160	34.5	100	2.2	1.9	7.6	524
Nutrison Standard	Nutricia	100	4.0	3.9	12.3	0	<0.02	82	0.7	80	1.6	1.2	5.7	315
Nutrison Multi-Fibre	Nutricia	100	4.0	3.9	12.3	1.5	<0.02	82	0.7	80	1.6	1.2	5.7	250

a. Nutrini and Nutrini Energy contains 0 g fibre/100 ml.
b. Paediasure and Paediasure Plus contains 0 g fibre/100 ml.
c. Tentrini and Tentrini Energy contains 0 g fibre/100 ml.

6. Semi-elemental formula

Product Name	Manu-facturer	MCT (%)	Nutritional composition per 100 ml												Osmolality (mOsmol/ kgH_2O)
			Energy (kcal)	Protein (g)	Fat (g)	Carb (g)	Fibre (g)	Lactose (g)	Vit A (μg RE)	Vit D (μg)	Calcium (mg)	Iron (mg)	Zinc (mg)	Selenium (μg)	
Infants 1–12 months of age															
Casein hydrolysate															
Nutra-migen 1	Mead Johnson	–	68	1.9	3.4	7.5	0	–	60	1.0	64	1.2	0.5	1.5	290
Nutra-migen 2 (from 6 months)	Mead Johnson	–	72	2.3	3.5	7.8	0	–	66	1.08	90	1.3	0.5	1.6	342
Pregestimil	Mead Johnson	54	68	1.9	3.8	6.9	0	–	77	1.25	78	1.2	0.7	1.5	330
Whey hydrolysate															
Pepti	Cow & Gate	–	66	1.6	3.6	6.8	0	2.6	64	1.5	52	0.5	0.5	1.2	240
Pepti-Junior	Cow & Gate	50	67	1.8	3.6	6.8	0	<0.1	77	1.3	54	0.9	0.4	1.3	190

6. Semi-elemental formula *contnued*

Product Name	Manu-facturer	MCT (%)	Nutritional composition per 100 ml												Osmolality (mOsmol/ kgH_2O)
			Energy (kcal)	Protein (g)	Fat (g)	Carb (g)	Fibre (g)	Lactose (g)	Vit A (µg RE)	Vit D (µg)	Calcium (mg)	Iron (mg)	Zinc (mg)	Selenium (µg)	
Non-milk derived peptides															
Pepdite	SHS	5	71	2.1	3.5	7.8	0	–	79	1.3	45	1.0	0.75	1.7	237
MCT Pepdite	SHS	75	68	2.0	2.7	8.8	0	–	79	1.3	45	1.0	0.75	1.7	290
Children above 1–10 years															
Peptamen Junior – whey hydro-lysate	Nestle	60	100	3.0	3.9	13.8	0	<0.2	45	1.0	91	1.0	1.0	3.0	310
Pepdite 1+ – non-milk derived peptides	SHS	35	100	3.1	3.9	13.0	0	–	86	0.6	56	1.1	1.1	3.4	465
Children above 6 years of age															
Peptisorb – whey hydro-lysate	Nutricia	< 1	100	4.0	1.7	17.6	0.1	0	82	0.7	80	1.6	1.2	5.7	535
Perative	Abbott	42	131	6.7	3.7	17.7	-	0	139	0.9	87	1.6	1.5	6.1	385

7. Elemental formula

Product Name	Manu-facturer	MCT (%)	Nutritional composition per 100 ml												Osmolality (mOsmol/ kgH_2O)
			Energy (kcal)	Protein (g)	Fat (g)	Carb (g)	Fibre (g)	Lactose (g)	Vit A (µg RE)	Vit D (µg)	Calcium (mg)	Iron (mg)	Zinc (mg)	Selenium (µg)	
Infants 1–12 months of age															
Neocate	SHS	5	71	2.0	3.5	8.1	0	–	79	1.3	49	1.1	0.75	1.7	360
Children aged 1–10 years															
Neocate Advance	SHS	35	100	2.5	3.5	14.6	0	–	37	0.8	50	0.6	0.5	2.5	610
Neocate Active Not suitable as sole source of nutrition	SHS	4	100	2.8	4.8	11.3	0	–	37	0.8	95	1.3	0.5	2.5	520
Children aged 5 years and above															
Elemental 028 Extra	SHS	35	89	2.5	3.5	11.8	0	–	66	0.5	49	0.8	0.8	3	502
Elemental 028 Extra Liquid flavoured	SHS	35	86	2.5	3.5	11	0	–	40	0.5	45	0.8	0.8	3	673–725

8. Vitamin and mineral supplements

Product name	Manu-facturer	Form	Suggested dosage	Nutritional composition per 100g									
				Energy (kcal)	Carb (g)	Calcium (mg)	Phosph (mg)	Magnes (mg)	Iron (mg)	Copper (mg)	Iodine (µg)	Zinc (mg)	Selenium (µg)
Paediatric Seravit available flavoured or un-flavoured	SHS	Powder	0– 6 months: 14g; 6–12 months: 17g; 1–7 years: 17–25g; 7–14 years: 25–35g *adjust depending on diet	300	75	2570	1714	357	69	4.6	332	46	137
				Vit A (µg RE)	Vit D (µg)	Vit E (mg αTE)	Vit C (mg)	Vit K (µg)	Thiamin (mg)	Niacin (mg)	Vit B6 (mg)	Folic (mg)	Vit B12 (µg)
				4200	55.5	21.4	400	166	3.2	35	3.4	303	8.6
Forceval	Alliance	Capsule	Child over 5 years: 2 capsules daily	Nutritional composition per capsule									
				Vit A (µg RE)	Vit D (µg)	Vit E (mg αTE)	Vit C (mg)	Vit K (µg)	Thiamin (mg)	Niacin (mg)	Vit B6 (mg)	Folic (mg)	Vit B12 (µg)
				375	5	5	25	25	1.5	7.5	1	100	2
				Energy (kcal)	Carb (g)	Calcium (mg)	Phosph (mg)	Magnes (mg)	Iron (mg)	Copper (mg)	Iodine (µg)	Zinc (mg)	Selenium (µg)
				-	-	-	-	1	5	1	75	5	25

9. Mineral supplements

A. Iron

Product name	Manufacturer	Form	Type of salt	Content
Ironorm Drops	Wallace	Oral drops	Ferrous sulphate	125 mg iron per 5 ml

B. Calcium

Product name	Manufacturer	Form	Type of salt	Content
Calcium-Sandoz	Alliance	Syrup	Calcium glubionate	108 mg calcium per 5 ml Calcium lactobionate
Sandocal-400 Sandocal-1000	Novartis Consumer Health	Effervescent	Calcium lactate gluconate Calcium cabonate	400 mg or 1000 mg per tablet
Cacit also available with Vitamin D (Cacit D3)	Procter & Gamble Pharmaceuticals	Effervescent	Calcium carbonate, disperses into calcium citrate when dissolved	500 mg per tablet

C. Zinc

Product name	Manufacturer	Form	Type of salt	Content
Solvazinc	Provalis	Effervescent	Zinc sulphate	45 mg per tablet

Appendix 6: Form for feeding and dietary assessment

This form has been designed for use by a dietitian. It can be used to collect information about a child's feeding in addition to the nutritional information obtained from a food diary or verbal diet history.

It can be adapted for use by other members of the multidisciplinary team, or the relevant parts filled in by members individually.

Date: **Name of child:** **Age:** **Interviewee:**

1. CLASSIFICATION OF DISABILITY
If child has cerebral palsy:
Spastic
Athetoid

Distribution of involvement

Hemiplegia
R/L
Diplegia
Tetraplegia
Triplegia

2. MOUTH
Speech difficulty

None
Some
Cannot talk
Communicates by signs

Drooling/dribbling
Continuous
Some of the time
Occasionally
Never
Wears a bib

3. MOBILITY
How well does the child walk?

Very well, no problem

Degree of disability:

Mild – can walk independently unaided
Moderate – can walk independently but sometimes needs help
Severe – always needs aids & helper to walk
Severe – cannot walk, needs a wheelchair

4. USE OF ARMS AND HANDS FOR FEEDING AND DRINKING
Assessment of self- feeding skills

Food
No difficulty, feeds self with one or both hands, no help required
Some difficulty
Needs help with feeding

Level of help required:
Always needs help
Some help needed e.g. hand over hand, chopping up of foods
Needs help towards end of meal as tires
Some meals can feed self, some meals needs help

What utensils are used by the child itself?
Knife
Fork
Spoon
Adapted cutlery
Adapted utensils

Does the child finger feed?
Yes
No

Right or left handed?
Right
Left

If child is fed by carer, what utensils are used?
Describe. . .. . .

Drink

No difficulty, able to hold cup etc., no help required

Some difficulty – need some help

Always needs help

What does the child use to give self a drink with?
Bottle
Adapted cup
Normal cup

What does the carer use to give the child a drink with?
Bottle
Adapted cup
Normal cup

4.SENSES

Sight	good	glasses	no useful vision	affects feeding
Hearing	good	impaired	hearing aids needed/worn	
Intellect	school /nursery – describe			
	Statemented? Y/N			

5. SWALLOWING AND FEEDING – 4 point scale of ability (Reilly et al 1996)[1] circle:

a. No apparent feeding problems, eats normal diet

b. Mild swallowing or feeding difficulty, requires chopped/mashed foods

c. Moderate swallowing or feeding difficulty and some difficulty with liquids. Requires well mashed or chopped food that is well moistened.

d. Severe difficulties with consuming liquids and foods, requires well moistened foods, thickened fluids, tube feeds etc.

6. MEDICATIONS
Name and amount:

How taken – mixed with food
On own
Tablets/ liquids

7. EATING PATTERNS OF FAMILY AND CHILD

Number in family home – adults and children

Meals and snacks eaten together as a family:

Weekdays	Weekends
Always/never	Always/never

Breakfast

Lunch

Evening meal

Snacks

Do you eat meals out as a family? Y/N

Where?

Does the child go as well?

Is the child fed on their own at all? Y/N

Why, where, when?

Do you cook and prepare food for child separately to rest of family? Y/N

Why is this?

How does the child's appetite and the amount they eat compare with siblings and peers?

Parent's/carers views on current nutritional status now . . . do they consider them adequately nourished?

What are the main problems (if any) that the parent/carers have feeding the child.

Does the child have particular food and drink preferences? If so, list . . .

Does the parent or carer avoid giving any specific foods/drinks to the child, and if so why?

How does child indicate they are?

Hungry –

Thirsty –

Have had enough to eat/drink –

Want a particular food/drink –

Does the child have opportunity to choose what they want to eat or drink?

Always sometimes never

24-hour dietary recall/normal daily intake (delete which).

Breakfast

Mid am

Lunch

Mid pm

Eve pm

Evening meal

Supper

Milk

Supplements/enteral feed

Other details:

Who feeds the child?

Is there a loss of food from mouth during feeding?

If so, how is this dealt with?

Duration of meals – minutes/hours – how long is spent feeding the child each day?

Supplements – micronutrients, calorie supplement, prescribable dietary supplements

Tooth cleaning/dental hygiene – oral aversion

What input with regard to feeding is there from?:
Occupational Therapy
Speech and Language Therapy
Physiotherapy
Play Therapy

Reference

1. Reilly JJ, Hassan TM, Braekken A, Jolly J, Day RE. Growth retardation and undernutrition in children with spastic cerebral palsy. *J Hum Nutr and Diet* 1996; 9: 429–35.

Index

Abbreviations: CP, cerebral palsy; FAQs, frequently asked questions.